The Essential Guide
to Running the
New York City
Marathon

The Essential Guide to Running the New York City Marathon

Toby Tanser

A PERIGEE BOOK

A Perigee Book
Published by the Berkley Publishing Group
A division of Penguin Putnam Inc.
375 Hudson Street
New York, New York 10014

First edition: February 2003

Visit our website at www.penguinputnam.com

Library of Congress Cataloging-in-Publication Data

Tanser, Toby.
The essential guide to running the New York City Marathon / Toby Tanser.
p. cm.
Includes index.
ISBN 0-399-52852-0
1. New York City Marathon, New York, N.Y.   2. Marathon running—Training.   I. Title.

GV1065.22.N49 T36 2003
796.42'52—dc21
2002030313

Printed in the United States of America

10 9 8 7 6 5 4 3 2 1

This book is dedicated to the people who take the most gruelling discipline in the Olympic calendar and have the courage to take on the challenge of running a marathon.
Having raced in five continents (over 500 races),
one race stands for me above all others!

Contents

Introduction   ix

Chapter One
Beginning Running   1

Chapter Two
**A Brief History of the
New York City Marathon**   9

Chapter Three
How to Enter the Marathon   21

Chapter Four
Training for the Marathon   31

Chapter Five
Where to Stay and Orientation   51

Chapter Six
Food in the City   81

Chapter Seven
Getting to the Start   97

Chapter Eight
**Spectating: Where to
Watch the Runners**   107

Chapter Nine
The Race   119

Chapter Ten
After the Marathon   135

Chapter Eleven
**Things to Do and Places
of Interest in New York**   143

Chapter Twelve
Facts and Figures   161

Resources   167
Index   179

Introduction

The marathon demands determination and courage. The event should not be taken lightly; it asks us to reach down and test our mettle; rise above our limits, to become more disciplined, and to make substantial sacrifices. The rewards are unique: a sense of achievement beyond the scope of words.

New York is the unofficial capital of the world, a city where millions of people's paths cross, and for many runners, the ultimate experience in marathoning is the New York City Marathon. All you need to know to enter, train for, and run this Marathon of Marathons is in this book—plus a runner-friendly guide to New York City.

It can be an intimidating experience. People ask themselves: Could I finish a marathon? My answer is: Go and watch a local race. You will see runners of all shapes, sizes, and ages complete the distance, and one thing unites them all: they were all once beginning runners. It has been said that it's a sin not to try new challenges, I believe that it is indeed vital to endeavor to improve ourselves, to

> "The marathon is the people's Everest."
>
> —Olympian Peter Fonseca

not only accept challenges as they present themselves, but to seek them out. Yes, a marathon is tough—but therein lies its merit. Go forth and conquer!

What Is the Marathon?

On what was presumably a scorching summer's day in 490 B.C., the legendary Greek foot-soldier Pheidippides ran twenty-four hilly miles from Marathon to Athens. He delivered the news that the Athenian Army had defeated the Persians. But the exertion of his long run had been too much, and Pheidippides fell dead from exhaustion shortly afterward.

This story was the inspiration for the sporting event that we call the marathon. Before the first modern Olympic Games of 1896, Michel Breal, a philologist at the Sorbonne, suggested that it would be fitting to include an event that commemorated the Pheidippides legend: a 24½-mile race from Marathon to Athens.

On April 10, 1896, the final day of the Games, twenty-five runners stood at the starting line by the Warriors' Tomb on the Plain of Marathon. Appropriately, the man who arrived first at the Olympic Stadium in Athens was a Greek. It had taken Spiridon Louis two hours, fifty-eight minutes, and fifty seconds to complete the distance. The twenty-three-year-old received a medal, a certificate, and a wreath of olive branches.

> "People were screaming for me the whole way! They are very encouraging, so nice to see."
>
> —Two-time NYC Marathon champion John Kagwe

It was not until the 1908 Olympics in London that the Marathon's 26.2-mile distance was standardized. Apparently, the Queen wanted the race to finish in front of the royal box; thus an extra 385 yards was added to the twenty-six miles!

Why the New York City Marathon?

As recently as the 1960s, runners who continued to train after their college years were considered cranks. The few available races, such as the Boston Marathon, were small-scale events that attracted a few hundred competitors at best.

Today there are literally hundreds of marathons. Virtually every major city in America, and at least one city in most countries throughout the world, puts on a marathon race; however, for many, New York will always remain *the* race to run.

A world-class field; more than 30,000 eager participants; more spectators than at any other one-day sporting event in the world; the excitement of running through all five boroughs of the world's most famous city; proven, reliable organization— all these ingredients make the New York City Marathon a special choice.

> "It gives you chills; no other marathon has given me the chills."
>
> —Tom Cheslik, finisher of more than fifteen marathons

What New York has done for the marathon can only be described as giving birth to marathon racing for the populace. One of the toughest disciplines on the Olympic agenda has been made popular for the masses. More than a half-million people have finished the marathon in Manhattan's Central Park.

When you combine the marathon experience with what else New York has to offer, you can have a truly marvelous marathon occasion— if you plan ahead, and utilize what the city has to offer. After an event that has taken a few months of training, you definitely deserve to celebrate—and for culture and entertainment, New York is nonpareil. Use this book to organize a running holiday that will be a memory for a lifetime.

The Essential Guide
to Running the

New York City
Marathon

Chapter One

Beginning Running

No matter why you start running—what your goals, desires, and purpose are—congratulations. Running is a simple, yet very effective way to improve your life.

The benefits are numerous. Running gives you a bigger set of lungs, a stronger heart, increased stamina, a leaner, toned physique . . . the list goes on. And on top of the physical gains, as a runner, you become an "I can" person who takes up challenges. The confidence built by achieving physical goals will carry over into many aspects of your life.

How do I start?

Running is a simple sport. Very little equipment is needed for running. You will need a good pair of running shoes, and some basic sports clothes. It is advisable to start any fitness program with a full medical checkup. Once your doctor has given you the go-ahead, you're ready to begin!

Running shoes

Go to a running specialist store—and if you have a friend who's an experienced runner, take him or her along with you. Running magazines frequently have shoe reviews; check the racks for such an article before you hit the stores.

TOP SHOE TIPS

▪ You need shoes designed specifically for running. Tennis shoes, basketball shoes, and even "cross-trainers" are second-class choices.

▪ Don't rush your purchase. Expect to take a good forty minutes to choose a pair of running shoes. They aren't a cheap item, and any salesperson worth buying from will expect you to to take your time and make an intelligent choice. Ask your salesperson if she's a runner. If she seems to know nothing about running, be wary!

▪ Visit the store in the afternoon, when your feet will be at their biggest. (Feet expand throughout the day.)

▪ Running shoes no longer take miles to break in. If a shoe feels wrong in the store, it probably isn't right for your foot.

▪ Run around the store, and even out in the street if the store allows it, to find out if you feel comfortable in the shoe, while it does its real job. Bring the socks that you most often use for running.

▪ There should be at least a half-inch of toe room. Your feet will swell slightly while you run.

▪ The shoe's heel should be firmly in place; it shouldn't move as you push off in a running stride.

▪ Try on a wide variety of shoes. Don't go for a certain brand just because it suits a friend; different brands—and models—fit different folks.

■ If you wear orthotics, bring them—and make sure that they work with the shoe that you choose. A good pair of running shoes will typically cost between $60 and $120.

■ To be on the safe side, ask about return policies.

Clothing

Man-made fibers, such as CoolMax (found in running stores), do work. Period. Running is far more enjoyable in quality clothes. Try to find shorts and shirts specifically designed for running—you'll reduce the chances of chafing and of restricted movement.

Once you're running, your body will generate heat. Keep this in mind when dressing to run; if you feel comfortable when you step outside on a cool or cold day, you'll probably be too warm for comfort after a couple of miles. However, remember that if you have overdressed, you can remove a layer, whereas underdressing can lead to a miserable experience! As the saying goes, "There's no such thing as bad weather, merely bad clothes."

58° F and above	Usually calls for a T-shirt and shorts
48–58° F	Sweatshirt and long tights
32–48° F	Add gloves and a hat
below 32° F	Insulated running jacket and pants, cold-weather socks, maybe mittens and a balaclava if there's wind

Once properly outfitted, head out to the park. If you have to run on the road, please watch out for the traffic.

First Steps

The cardinal rule of the new runner is *be patient*. Your body needs time to adapt to this new activity that you're asking it to perform. It may be uncomfortable at first, but you'll begin to see results fairly quickly. All the same, it's important to build *gradually*.

12 TIPS FOR BEGINNERS

- Once again, be patient

- Stretch before and after you run

- Don't hesitate to alternate running and walking at any time in your program

- Start and finish each run at a slow pace

- Run more slowly than you think you can

- Don't run as far as you think you can

- Don't be overly concerned with running form; often your natural form is the best

- Try to run relaxed

- Aim for consistency with your program

- Try to make running friends, and ask them for advice if you're in doubt

- Reward yourself; for example, buy a new piece of running gear for each completed week of training

- Remember that running should always be fun. (Well, almost always.)

Beginners' Running Program

This schedule should help the absolute beginner to advance to a stage where he can call himself a runner.

WEEK ONE   Alternate 3 days of exercise with 4 days of rest.
    21 minutes of walking for 2 minutes, jogging for 1 minute

WEEK TWO   3 days of 24 minutes: walking 2 minutes, jogging 1 minute

WEEK THREE   3 days of 28 minutes: walking 2 minutes, jogging 2 minutes

WEEK FOUR   3 days of 35 minutes: walking 2 minutes, jogging 3 minutes
    We now switch from the term *jogging* to *running*. Don't worry about your speed at all, just run how you feel!

WEEK FIVE   3 days of 35 minutes: walking 1:30 and running 3:30.

WEEK SIX   First day of the 3-day week: 2 × 10 minutes running with 2 minutes walking
    Second day: 2 × 15 minutes running and 3 minutes walking
    Third day: 25 minutes of continuous running

WEEK SEVEN   3 alternating days of 30-minute continuous runs

WEEK EIGHT   3 alternating days of 35-minute continuous runs

    Now try adding a fourth day of running each week. If you're running on more days than you're not running—you must be a runner! Well done.

Now What?

Be careful not to try to increase your mileage too fast—that's a sure-fire way to pick up an injury. Consistency is the key to any running program. Don't increase your mileage by more than 10 percent each week, and don't try to increase it every single week. You might consider dropping your mileage 10 percent on every third week to ensure that the body can cope with the demands of an increasingly challenging training program.

After a few months of consistency, you may decide that you want to take your running to the next level.

Your First Race

Why not be a spectator at your first race? Watch not only the fastest but also the slowest runners. Stand at the finish line and soak up their sense of achievement. Then join them.

Your goal for the first race that you run should be just to complete the course. Set off with caution, and don't get caught up in any other runner's pace. You should find a very supportive, communal, and enjoyable community around you, both in the field and along the course. This sport is peopled by very friendly, very social participants; enjoy the other runners, and have a great time—without caring about the time on the clock.

Anxieties, Worries, and Doubts!

While training for a marathon, you'll definitely get some sore muscles—and you might pick up an injury along the way. But you can minimize the risks. A runner becomes a scrupulous inspector of her body, until she can tell a simple ache because of sleeping in an unusual position from a "running niggle." Basically, no one's body is prepared to run 26.2 miles. You must train your body to be able to cover such a distance. Along the way, soreness will be a reminder that you are a runner, and fatigue is common, too. British Olympian Brendan Foster once said that a distance runner goes to bed tired, and he wakes up tired, too!

"The Marathon is a charismatic event. It has everything. It has drama. It has competition. It has camaraderie. It has heroism. Every jogger can't be an Olympic champion, but can dream of finishing a marathon."

—Fred Lebow, founder; five-borough NYC Marathon

If an injury does strike, don't panic; it doesn't mean that your running is over. Often a day of rest, or two, will clear up the problem. Most marathon plans will not be 100 percent completed. That's okay, even expected. If you cover most of a marathon training plan, you'll succeed in finishing the marathon. More on marathon training can be found in Chapter 4.

Chapter Two

A Brief History of
the New York City Marathon

On September 13, 1970, Gary Muhrcke was presented with a wrist-watch for winning the inaugural New York City Marathon. Muhrcke, who paid a $1 entry fee, had completed a little more than four loops of Manhattan's Central Park to defeat the other 127 starters. Fifty-five men, and no women, made it to the finish line.

The following year, Beth Bonner would win the women's division in 2:55:22, becoming the first woman to officially break the three-hour barrier.

Another year later in 1972, the women again broke ground as they refused to start ten minutes before the men's event as required by the Amateur Athletic Union. The Union responded by adding ten minutes to the times of all the female finishers. A court case later ruled in favor of the women, and the times were readjusted.

By 1973 the race had acquired a hint of professionalism: The men's winner, Tom Fleming, was awarded an around-the-globe air ticket. Recalls Fleming, "It was a small race then. Running in the park wasn't bad, as we did not talk about 'fast course' so much back then."

Hot weather caused a record 40 percent of the field to drop out of the race in 1974. This would never happen today, as runners are better prepared for the rigors of the marathon. Kathrine Switzer, one of the founders of women's distance running, took first place. She remembers,

The 1974 New York City Marathon was my first big attempt to go under three hours, and I was totally ready. I was so ready that I refused to even think about the fact that it was something like ninety-five degrees with high humidity. When I went out at a sub-3:00 pace, I was right behind the lead guys. Pretty soon everybody began falling by the wayside and it seemed I was running with nobody, passing a few, never being passed myself, but realizing I was slowing, slowing, and couldn't help it. Finally, going up the 110th Street hill for the last time [Remember, it was four laps!] the heavens opened, lightning cracked and thunder boomed, and I thought it was the end of the world. I vaguely thought that I shouldn't be out there like a lightning rod, but I didn't care anymore if I died, I was going to run the hell out of that race if it killed me, since I'd trained so much of my life for it.

Kathrine would go on, running in ankle-deep water, to win by twenty-seven minutes and fourteen seconds, the largest margin ever. In her next marathon, she smashed the three-hour barrier.

The following year was the last time the marathon would be held inside Central Park, and fittingly, Kim Merritt and Tom Fleming ran course records of 2:46:14 and 2:19:27 respectively. Fleming thus remains the only man in history to run a sub-2:20 marathon in Central Park. "I was prouder of a thirty-kilometer race I ran in 1:30 in the park," he says now, "but yes, it was a very tough course to run."

A logistical phenomenon was achieved in 1976. One must remember that at this time marathon running had not reached the lofty status it holds today. With a paltry 534 entrants having entered the race in the previous year, Fred Lebow still managed to convince city officials to close major roads for hours to let him thread the course through New York's unique five boroughs—a race organizer's nightmare.

Bill Rodgers, one of America's finest marathoners ever, came, saw, and won the event in a world-class time of 2:10:10. The New York City Marathon had arrived on the international scene.

The 1977 race featured repeat winners: Rodgers and Miki Gorman, who ran 2:43:10 at age 42. As runners crossed the finish line, volunteers handed out Mylar blankets for the first time. Many a runner has since been thankful for these silver "warmth" blankets. With 4,821 entrants, the New York City Marathon had become the largest in the world.

A world record was set in New York in 1978. Grete Waitz, a Norwegian schoolteacher who trained at 5 A.M. each day, but who had never run a road race, turned in a sterling time of 2:32:30, shattering the world record by over two minutes, and then vowed never to run the distance again. (Famous first words!) Bill Rodgers took the hat trick with his third straight win.

Both Rodgers and Waitz won again in 1979 as the event truly became global: Athletes from fifty-six different countries entered. The amazing Grete smashed her own world record—and the 2:30 barrier—with her 2:27:33. (At this time, the longest running event for women in the Olympic Games was slightly *less than one mile*, due to archaic views about the stamina of women.) Performance-related prize money was awarded for the first time; under-the-table appearance money had previously been paid to some top runners, but now the event became a pioneer in taking road running into the professional era. The field had now grown to more than 10,000.

In 1980, Alberto Salazar, from Oregon, came to the race with the bold prediction that he would break 2:10 in his first marathon. He did, setting a new course record of 2:09:41. It was the fastest-ever debut for a marathoner. Not to be outdone, Waitz lowered her own world record to 2:25:42.

Marathon running, globally, was now moving into the big leagues. Realizing its growing popularity, ABC television aired the race nationally for the first time. It was a good year to televise the NYC Marathon, as Salazar and Allison Roe of New Zealand ran what were then thought to be world records. (Remeasurements of the course revealed that the distance was slightly short.) Nevertheless, the top runners in the world were choosing New York City as the event to run. In third place was British Olympian Hugh Jones, who would later win the prestigious London Marathon. He recalls of the event,

> I'd only just come a good five months earlier by winning the Triple-A Marathon at Rugby [A small English town], and I was still wide-eyed at the prospect of what might follow. New York was my first big-city race, but the experience was predigested from reading and hearing reports of it. I knew the city from previous visits, although the last time had been six years before. In retrospect, it's amazing how seamlessly one can transfer from sixty competitors around the back roads of Rugby to fifteen thousand up the main roads of Manhattan. After all, the central question is performance, not where the performance is enacted.

Chiseling his name forever into the history of the event, Alberto Salazar returned in 1982 to become the second man in the race's short history to win three in a row. Grete Waitz, sidelined the previous year with injuries, returned to the streets of New York and took another title.

In 1983, Rod Dixon of New Zealand became the event's first non-American male winner. Dixon chased down a British fireman, Geoff Smith, in Central Park to win by seven seconds. Smith broke Salazar's marathon debut record. Grete Waitz was again the winner.

Mercedes-Benz became an event sponsor in 1984. The prize money was negligible compared to the $25,000 luxury sedans awarded by the auto manufacturer to the men's and women's winners. Orlando Pizzolato of Italy and Grete Waitz became the lucky drivers.

The race's 100,000th finisher crossed the line in 1985, the fifteenth running. The winners from 1984 repeated.

Numbers were escalating. The 1986 race had more than 20,000 entrants! Eighty countries were represented. Another Italian, Gianni Poli, took the men's title, and there were three more Italians in the top eight. Grete Waitz cemented her position as the ruling monarch of the New York roads with her eighth victory.

New York had an uncanny knack of making athletes' names, almost in the same way that Broadway does with actors. In 1987, two more legends surfaced: Ibrahim Hussein and Priscilla Welch. Ibrahim, a shy Kenyan studying in America, became the first African to win a big-city marathon. "I am very proud to be the first African to win the New York City Marathon. I found the city nice to run in, flat . . . I do not think New York is a tough course at all. Boston is a much harder course," he remarked. Priscilla was in the British army and had been a smoker into her thirties. Now aged 42, she won in a masters' record of 2:30:17 that still stands.

The military vein ran into the next year's event when a British Air Force officer destroyed the field with a fabulous 2:08:20 performance. Steve Jones, a former world record–holder, ran what was then the second-fastest performance ever on New York's roads—just seven seconds behind Salazar's 2:08:13 on the short course!

Grete Waitz won her ninth title, and it was to be her last. The field had now grown to 23,463; due to the ever-increasing numbers, both decks of the Verrazano-Narrows Bridge were used.

*   *   *

Perfect weather produced fast running in 1989. A course record was set by yet another military officer when Major Juma Ikangaa of Tanzania soloed a 2:08:01 national record. Norway's other famous female runner, the then-world record-holder Ingrid Kristiansen, took the honors, running 2:25:30—one second slower than Roe's short-course record.

The 1990 race was dedicated to the race director, Fred Lebow, who had been afflicted with brain cancer. Lebow can rightly be called the father of the modern marathon. It is impossible to calculate the immense impact that he had upon the marathon as a marketable event. Wanda Panfil became Poland's first winner, and in the men's division Douglas Wakiihuri of Kenya won. "Winning New York was important for my career. Many Kenyans hold this event higher than the Olympic silver I won in 1988," Wakiihuri recounted years later.

Another record was set in 1991 when Liz McColgan, from Britain, won with the fastest-ever female debut marathon. It was less than one year since she had given birth to her daughter Eilish. The Hispanic quarter of the city had reason to celebrate when Salvador García of Mexico won the men's division, and he delighted fans by accepting his award dressed in national attire—complete with sombrero.

Fred Lebow somehow managed to run the marathon in 1992. The sixty-year-old was accompanied every step of the way by Grete Waitz. The crowds waited in the rain to salute Fred, who finished in 5:32:34. An unknown South African Zulu tribesman named Willie Mtolo won the race in the first year that South Africans were allowed to compete outside their country. Lisa Ondieki, a former 400-meter hurdler from Australia, blasted a new course record of 2:24:40.

*   *   *

In 1993, a very determined Mexican toed the line. Andres Espinosa had been the runner-up for the previous two editions of the New York City Marathon, and he had resorted to sticking a Mercedes emblem on the front of his Volkswagen Jetta back home in Mexico to symbolize the car that was awarded to the race's winner! Espinosa remembers, "New York is bigger to Mexicans than it is even to New Yorkers. I really wanted to win." He did, breaking away from American Bob Kempainen in the twenty-third mile.

Making her New York debut after attending a training camp in Boulder, Colorado, was a German lady who would become a marathon legend, Uta Pippig. She blazed a 1:11 first half to distance herself from a strong field and won in 2:26:14, a glorious time for the unseasonably hot conditions the runners faced that year.

In an attempt to drum up a stronger American challenge, the race offered double prize money for the first five places. Two Americans were able to capitalize on this bonus, Kempainen (2nd) and Keith Brantly (5th).

A somber shadow was cast when, four weeks before the 1994 run, Fred Lebow died of brain cancer. It was the silver jubilee edition, and it became famous for an incident concerning a man named Silva.

Two Mexicans ran in front, side by side, in the race's late stages. Then, on Central Park South, a break was made. German Silva moved a few yards ahead of his compatriot Benjamin Paredes—and then followed a press vehicle off the course! Paredes moved ahead, but was quickly chased down, and defeated, by the man now known as "Wrong-Way Silva."

A tiny Kenyan girl named Tegla Chepkite Loroupe made her marathon debut in this race. The previous year, she had finished fourth in the World Championships at 10,000 meters. She became the first African woman winner of a big-city marathon, emulating the performance of her countryman, Ibrahim Hussein, in 1987. She inspired a nation of Kenyan women.

A statue of Fred Lebow, which today stands along the course in Central Park, was unveiled to honor the father of the modern marathon.

Allan Steinfeld, who had taken over as the race director in 1994, had been with the NYRR club since the early sixties. An accomplished runner with 22-second 200-meter credentials, he left no doubt that the show would go on, even without Mr. Lebow. The 1995 men's race produced a repeat winner when Silva managed to pull away from Paul Evans, a tough Englishman who hadn't started running until the relatively late age of 27. Silva waited on the finishing line to congratulate the women's winner—Tegla Loroupe, another returning victor. Loroupe's elder sister, Albina, had died in the week prior to the race, and this made the marathon a very emotional battle for the tearful Pokwot tribeswoman.

It was fitting that the Romanian national record was set in the 1996 race when a countrywoman of the late Fred Lebow won the race and dedicated the win to his memory. Anuta Catuna (the only winner with a palindromic name) reeled in the fast-starting Loroupe, who faded to seventh.

An overlooked Italian put in two of the fastest closing miles ever and stole the men's race. A select field of East Africans was expected to dominate the field, and indeed, they took six of the top ten spots—but Giacomo Leone, who had been inspired by the Italian wins of the 80's, would rule New York City for a day.

A pair of brand-new Nike racing shoes gave John Kagwe the win in 1997, but they may have cost him the course record. Kagwe, a Kenyan who confessed to having hated running as a youngster, picked up the new shoes at the exposition a couple of days prior to the race. Thus they were not really tried and tested—a cardinal running sin. The laces came undone three times in the final few miles, and twice John stopped to tie them. His winning time was a scintillating 2:08:12, twelve seconds away from breaking the course record.

Lawyer, restaurateur, and national record-holder Franziska Rochat-Moser of Switzerland gave her country its first New York win when she flew by Tegla Loroupe in the closing miles to take a surprise victory in 2:28:43. Sadly, Rochat-Moser died in the spring of 2002 while vacationing in the Alps.

Persistence paid off for Franca Fiacconi in 1998. Her singlet covered in sponsors' logos, the tall Italian finally captured a NYCM title. She had first run the race in 1992 and finished twelfth; her next two attempts, in 1996 and 1997, had put her on the podium. Now she took control of her own fate by dictating the pace and storming to a clear win. Fiacconi delighted reporters by saying that winning the event was the best thing that had ever happened to her.

John Kagwe prevailed in the race's closest three-man finish ever as he held off countryman Joseph Chebet and Tanzanian Zebedayo Bayo to take his second title. A mere six seconds covered the trio, and the Kenyans had six runners in the top ten places. Two-time winner German Silva ran his fastest New York City Marathon and placed only fourth.

The ChampionChip was put into play for the 1999 edition of the marathon. This ingenious device, invented by a cattle farmer, gave the race organizers a reprieve at the finishing funnels as electronic automatic timing clocked all the finishers via a tiny chip attached to each runner's shoe.

Patrick Sang, an Olympic steeplechase medalist, had this to say of Joseph Chebet an hour before the 1999 race: "He'll win the race. He has trained the hardest—no one could've trained harder." Rather like Andres

Espinosa in 1993, Chebet was tired of his runner-up positions. "People in Kenya were saying I could not win!" he said. (They were wrong.)

Adriana Fernandez, coached by two-time runner-up Rodolfo Gomez, became a heroine in her country as the first Mexican female to win a big-city marathon. Battling tough headwinds, she ran the majority of the race all alone—odd, since 30,000 runners were sharing the roads with her. Catherine Ndereba, then a little-known Kenyan girl, made her marathon debut, finished second, and fell in love with the marathon event. "The people cheered and cheered for me. It was wonderful!" (Catherine would claim the marathon world record in the fall of 2001.)

The millennium edition saw Russia claim her first individual title. Ludmila Petrova, a former Olympian at 10,000 meters who was running her second New York City Marathon, pushed the pace in the final few miles to break away from Kenyan Margaret Okayo, who was then passed by Franca Fiacconi. However, the Kenyan women had begun to show the dominance that the Kenyan men had been exhibiting on the streets of New York: Five of them finished in the top ten. Abdelkhader El Mouaziz complained, "The pacemakers were unable to keep the pace—I had to go alone . . . early." And go he did, scorching the first half of the course in just over 1:03! Although he faded badly in Central Park, the Moroccan could not be caught. Mouaziz, like Petrova, put a new flag on the winners' rostrum.

In 2001, the Marathon was New York City's first major event following the terrorist attacks of September 11. The city came together under a "United We Run" banner, and race director Steinfeld commented, "Never before have I seen so many American flags out there." There was never any doubt that the marathon would be held, though many wondered if people would stay away from the city in fear of further attacks. The concern was allayed as thousands poured into the city to show global support for New York.

Beautiful weather and a slightly altered course rewarded the race organizers with two new course records. Tesfaye Jifar, with his 2:07:43, became the first Ethiopian to win the event, and Margaret Okayo of Kenya stormed ahead after the halfway point to run unchallenged to a 2:24 victory.

Jifar, who lost one eye in a childhood farming accident, followed a duo of Kenyans until the 22-mile mark, when he attacked fiercely. "I like to follow so I can see where the opponents are," he explained to journalists, who wondered why he had run behind the Kenyans for so long. "But yes, I was fresh; I could have pushed ahead for a faster time if I wanted."

Okayo had had the dubious honor of losing the Chicago Marathon in 1999 by a mere second when countrywoman Joyce Chepchumba sprinted past her. With Chepchumba again in the field, Okayo wasn't taking any chances. At the twelve-mile point, she pushed hard to distance herself from the pack, and on Fifth Avenue she ran a super-fast 5:07 mile to leave the other women fighting for second place.

The Marathon Before the Marathon

The New York City Marathon takes momentous amounts of planning. The New York Road Runners work year round to produce the event. A week after the 2001 event, Race Director Allan Steinfeld was certainly not taking a holiday. "We have meetings, sponsors to talk to and thank, bills to be paid, checks to be written . . ." he explained.

The élite field of the marathon is put together months before the race by New Yorker David Monti. David decides how much appearance money the top athletes will be offered, and

ESTIMATED ECONOMIC IMPACT OF THE NEW YORK CITY MARATHON

$118,128,000 (2001)

Source: NYRR

then he coordinates invitations, visas, and the care of the athletes and their managers in New York.

ATHLETE INTERVIEW
Margaret Okayo, Course Record-Holder

Q: *How does it feel to not only win but be the fastest ever on the streets of New York?*
MO: Very good. I trained very hard for this race.

Q: *After being beaten in last year's race, did you change your tactics?*
MO: In 2000 I was tripped. This year I decided to run away early from the pack. I decided to go at halfway.

Q: *Were you surprised to get the course record?*
MO: No, I knew I could run the course record. But I am very, very happy. Oh, my goodness, to win here is a blessing!

Q: *What are you going to do with your winnings?*
MO: Invest back home in Kenya.

Q: *Do you want to run this race again?*
MO: Yes—I want to *win* this race again!

Chapter Three

How to Enter the Marathon

Every year, approximately 70,000 people apply to run the NYC Marathon. Due to the logistics of the city, the size of the roads, and other factors, only about 30,000 can be accepted to run each year. This is divided into approximately 10,000 international runners and 20,000 domestic runners, giving a unique global ambiance to the race.

Strolling around the race exposition, or expo, in the three days before the race and watching the International Friendship Run the day before the marathon, one can easily see the delight in this multinational equation.

There are a few ways to enter.

Lottery

The most common is through a lottery, a process made simple by an online application available on the nycmarathon.org website. Applications for the lottery are also accepted through the mail. An application can be requested by writing to:

NYRR
Attn: NYC Marathon entry-form request
9 East 89th Street
New York, NY 10128

The submissions must be made online, or sent, before June 1. A nonrefundable processing fee of $7 is charged.

The Wheelchair and Hand-Crank Divisions

In the year 2000, the NYRR introduced official divisions for wheelchairs and hand-crank-propelled chairs. The race starts approximately thirty minutes ahead of the main field, due to safety concerns. The lead chair-racers fly around the course in times well under two hours.

In 2001, cash prizes were offered for these divisions and the race attracted a stellar field. These athletes train similar distances to the top runners—up to 130 miles per week. The hand-crank cyclist should, on paper, defeat the wheelchair athlete, and the respective course records reflect this:

COURSE RECORDS

Wheelchair		Hand Crank	
Women	Francesca Porcellato, 2:11:57, 2001	Women	Helene Hines, 1:46:22, 2001
Men	Krige Schabort, 1:38:27, 2002	Men	Franz Nietlispach, 1:26:57, 2002

Wheelchair and hand-crank competitors should contact the NYRR for a special entry form, which must be submitted before August 1 of the year prior to the race. Request the "For Athletes with Disabilities" form.

NYRR Race Participation

New York–area runners (and determined travelers) can secure guaranteed entry by running a predetermined number of NYRR-organized races (currently nine) in the year prior to the marathon, although they must also be paid members of the NYRR for the entire qualifying year.

Qualifying Times

Time standards for guaranteed entry have recently been introduced: If you've run under these times on a USATF- or AIMS-certified course, you're in!

	Marathon	Half-Marathon
Open Men	2:45:00	1:16:00
Open Women	3:15:00	1:31:00
Masters (40+) Men	3:00:00	1:24:00
Masters Women	3:30:00	1:39:00

The times for 40-and-over runners apply to age at the qualifying race, not on the day of the New York City Marathon.

Proof of a qualifying time must be submitted with the entry form before May 1 of the year of the event. A qualifying time in a marathon must have been achieved within the two years before the New York City Marathon; the period is shorter for half-marathon qualifiers. Contact the NYRR for the exact period.

Race Veterans

Those who have completed 15 or more past NYC Marathons are guaranteed an entry.

Fourth-Try Guaranteed Entry

The organizers have also introduced a clause that allows guaranteed entry for anyone who has been rejected by the lottery for the last three years. Says Gary Meltzer of the NYRR, "Basically, we want to make sure everyone has a way to get an entry to the marathon."

Guaranteed Entry Through Authorized Tour Operator

Guaranteed entry may be available along with the purchase of a package (at a minimum, entry and airfare) through an authorized tour operator in your country. The list of official tour operators becomes available in January of the marathon year. ENTRY ONLY IS NOT AVAILABLE. Residents of countries in which tour operators are available may select either the lottery or tour-operator option; the lottery is the only option for residents of countries without tour operators.

You must be eighteen years of age on the day of the race to run the NYC Marathon.

If All Goes Wrong

The New York City Marathon provides a deferral service that allows a runner to cancel by sending in his/her acceptance card, *postmarked before the marathon race day*. A guaranteed entry will be allotted to the runner should he/she apply for the following year's event.

ATHLETE PROFILE:
Joyce Chepchumba

Joyce has finished third, fourth, and fifth in the New York City Marathon. Despite having won the London and Chicago marathons twice apiece, Joyce really wants to win in New York. "Yes, it is a very special race. I love the people of New York, and the course is never boring," she says. Joyce emphasizes the importance of a good crowd. "In many smaller marathons, there are times when your focus goes, and you slow without realizing it. The crowds and their shouting keep you on course to run the best here."

So what does an elite athlete like Joyce do while she's in New York? Let's follow her through the week before and after the race.

TUESDAY: Joyce leaves her training base in Detmold, Germany. She has been training here for most of the year, sharing an apartment with her countrywoman Tegla Loroupe, the former world record-holder.

WEDNESDAY: She arrives at the Hilton Hotel in New York, and rests from the transatlantic trip. She drinks lots of water, and reads all the race information.

THURSDAY: She goes for a forty-minute run in Central Park on the dirt trails at a pace two and a half minutes per mile slower than she hopes to run in the race. After the run, she stretches a little. In the afternoon, she shops for clothes on 7th Avenue. In the evening she goes out looking for a pasta restaurant. "I like to eat plain food in the days before a marathon, but after traveling so much [Joyce has competed on six different continents!] I can eat almost anything."

FRIDAY: A rest day from running to revitalize the body and make sure she's fresh for Sunday's race. As one of the invited athletes, Joyce must attend a press conference, and a photo-shoot follows. She goes next to Niketown on 57th Street to buy some souvenirs for her friends back in Kenya, "and I need also some socks for myself for the race." Tourist chores are next: Joyce goes to the Empire State Building for the view of the city. She gets an hour-long massage at the hands of New York's marathon masseur, Harold Achille. In the evening, she goes out to Pasta d'Oro on 7th Avenue and eats a large plate of tortellini. A salad comes with the meal, but Joyce pushes it aside. "That is food for rabbits," she claims.

SATURDAY: Back to Central Park in the morning for a 40-minute run at the same pace as Thursday's. Some gentle stretching and a massage follow. Joyce is concerned about a pain in her hamstring that caused her to miss a week's training a month ago and has given her problems in her marathon-preparation period. The day is spent lazing around the hotel and chatting with athletes such as Susan Chepkemei and Esther Kiplagat. Pasta d'Oro is again the restaurant. The waiters whisper, "Look, that must be Tegla's sister."

SUNDAY: The race is on. Joyce runs at the back of the lead group, makes a mid-race challenge and moves up to second, but in the final few miles slips to fourth. She finishes in 2:25, and is happy with the result. "Not bad; the training was not good at all for this race," comments the Olympic marathon medalist.

Joyce sleeps for a couple of hours before going to the awards ceremony. Afterward she returns to Pasta d'Oro, but tonight she celebrates with some red wine.

MONDAY: A shopping day. The entire day is spent buying clothes for relatives and her nine-year-old son, Collins, who lives back in Kenya. Most of the shopping is done along 7th Avenue. The second-place woman, Susan Chepkemei, and the third-place man, Rodgers Rop, also come along. Rodgers haggles with the store owners over the prices as he would in his native Kenyan village; New York has been his debut marathon. Susan is impressed by the good quality yet reasonable prices offered in the New York clothing stores. Although she has won the Rotterdam Marathon, she believes that her runner-up spot in New York is a better result. "New York is . . . New York!" She laughs.

> "The crowds were awesome. Amazing. It was fantastic to run here. I've never seen anything like it!"
>
> —American national champion Deena Drossin

TUESDAY: Joyce's last day in New York before flying back to Germany and then on to Kenya. She buys two suitcases and some rubbing liniments for her legs. Then it's back to the Hilton for a buffet lunch. "After the marathon, I am trying to put on some kilos. I want to be big for Christmas!" she explains, half in jest.

WEDNESDAY: The flight home is spent in slumber. She will rest for a month back in Kenya before gradually returning to training, with a spring marathon in mind.

Volunteering

If you're going to be in New York, and you're not running the race, there's another way to participate. Why not sign up as a volunteer? More than 12,000 people help to make the event run smoothly before, while, and after the race is run. There are various ways that you can help.

Bus Loaders
For the early birds who want to do their bit before the race, and then spectate. Help is needed getting the runners on the buses to the start.

Water Station Workers
It takes a lot of volunteers to hand cups, and more cups, of water to the runners. This can be a wet job, but the thanks make it worth it.

Finish-Line Workers
Volunteers are needed to clip off the ChampionChips and to hand out Mylar blankets and finishers' medals. This is perhaps the most rewarding of all the volunteer positions—a virtual tidal wave of human emotion from the first to the last runner.

Baggage-Truck Crew
Very important people. They load up before the race then help find people's bags afterward.

Family Reunion Helpers
Runners are often a bit confused after running 26.2 miles, and they can use a little help locating family or friends at the reunion area. A smattering of languages comes in handy here.

Other volunteer jobs include number and T-shirt hand-out, goody-bag distribution, foreign-language translation, pasta-party ticket-taking . . . the list is near-endless! Contact the NYRR (www.nyrrc.org) a few months before the race if you'd like to volunteer. Spaces fill up quickly!

The Race Expo

In the days leading up to most major running races there is an exposition, usually called the "expo." It's a way for people in the commercial side of the running world to exhibit running products and to advertise upcoming races. Exhibitors rent booths to display their products; shoe companies often bring in celebrity runners to meet and talk to the public, and free samples are plentiful!

The New York City Marathon Exposition is currently held at the Jacob K. Javits Convention Center from the Wednesday to the Saturday before the race. It opens in the morning and closes as late as 8:00 P.M. (Check your acceptance package for the exact times.) The event is free, and it's also open to the general public. Free shuttle buses run to and from midtown Manhattan for your convenience.

The distribution of the race packages for all of the athletes takes place at the same site as the expo. Runners must bring photo identification along with their acceptance cards—no exceptions.

There are more than 300 booths at the expo, and their staffs will all be vying for your attention. Beware of trying unfamiliar foods, or types of massage, at the expo; the final days before a marathon are not a good time for experiments. The golden rule for the expo is to avoid staying on your feet for too long and tiring yourself out. Decide how long you'd be comfortable spending on your feet at the expo, and then stick to that time period. Too many runners wander from booth to booth for hours the day before the race, only to wake up on race day with aching calf muscles feeling like they've run their marathon at the expo.

EXPO TIPS

- Aim to pick up your race packet and not to spend too much time on your feet

- Take bottled water to keep hydrated

- Don't forget your photo ID or your registration acceptance card

- Take some money to buy some marathon souvenirs

- Eat well before you go; that way you won't be tempted to snack on sample food

Chapter Four

Training for the Marathon

Joseph Kimani sat bewildered and dehydrated. "I don't understand it," he lamented. "I can run 27:04 for ten-K, but today I felt like walking. My legs were not there!" The world-class Kenyan had just run a decidedly non-world-class 2:25 in the 1998 Boston Marathon.

Ask a running friend about one of his marathons, and the reply will probably be much more graphically elaborated than a simple finishing time and a date. Ask the same friend to describe his last two birthdays, and the vague reply will probably help you to understand the magic that imbues this running event.

The principles for running marathons are simple: getting used to running on tired legs, whether you're trying for a 2:07 or a 5:07. The mileage is just lower for the novice. Chances are, you already have an idea of how fast you want to try to run in your next marathon. If it will be your first, then use the old method of multiplying your most recent 10-kilometer time by 4.11.

Anyone interested in running a successful marathon—at any level—can learn from, and be inspired by, advice from people who have reached the highest levels of all. Here are a few such lessons:

The most important element in marathon running is that you absolutely must want to do it. Dutch 2:10 marathoner Greg Van Hest puts the message across eloquently: "First you have to love running; then the rest will easily follow."

Be realistic, and don't be afraid to reassess your marathon pace. Irish 2:22 marathoner Catherina McKiernan runs a shorter race a few weeks before a marathon. The result helps her to know if she should reevaluate her pace goal.

Don't become obsessed with long, *long* distance. Before Paul Evans's second-place finish in the 1995 New York City Marathon, he hadn't run for longer than one hour and thirty minutes in several months.

Paul Kipkoech, Kenya's first world track champion, often used to run a "flying kilometer" at faster-than-race speed a couple of times per week.

Non-running days help strengthen the body. While Steven Langat of Kenya trained to defend his Istanbul marathon title, his wife fell ill. Traveling home and attending to household duties left Langat training just four days a week, instead of the usual seven, throughout his whole three-month training period. He retained his title and ran a faster time than he had the year before.

"Use a well-worn uniform, and avoid spicy foods in the days before the race," offers USA national marathon team runner Eddy Hellebuyck.

Maria de Trujillo recommends that if it is your first marathon, "Take an easy pace, finish, and have a good feeling of accomplishment at the end."

Keep things in perspective. Doug Kurtis, the man who has recorded the most sub-2:20 marathons in history, has a timely reminder: "Remember to have fun. A marathon is a great achievement." Quite simply, if you're not having fun and enjoying your training, then stop, take a time-out, and plan for a later race.

Sessions of running at marathon pace are fundamental to finishing in one piece. Remember to be specific! Tanzania's Juma Ikangaa, NYC Marathon winner and course-record setter, often ran a workout in which he would begin at race pace and run for as long as he could at that speed. "If Tanzanians trained like I used to, we would be matching the Kenyans in marathon running. You must train at the pace you want to race at!" commands Major Ikangaa.

"Be patient, drink plenty," warns 2:09 marathoner Jerry Lawson.

"Training is the everyday work—then the race will be the holiday," says Zebedayo Bayo, another fast Tanzanian—third place in the 1998 NYC Marathon.

"Look at the weather on the morning of the race. . . Before Tokyo (World Championships, 1991) I was in my best form, but the high humidity killed my racing plans," says Swedish 2:10 marathoner Åke Erikson.

"Check your watch often, and run according to your race plan, not according to how you feel. It is better to go too slow at the start and finish strong than maybe not finish at all." This is the sage advice of Boston Marathon winner Amby Burfoot.

> "When I ran New York I forgot my own name. I underestimated the game. I came better prepared the next time."
>
> —Kenyan national marathon record-holder (2:06:16) Moses Tanui

The Training

Let's take a look at some of the challenges of a marathon:

- To run 26.2 miles, your cardiovascular system must be able to pump fuel to the muscles much more efficiently than a non-athlete's can.

- Several hours of running on unforgiving asphalt will cause a lot of jarring. Safeguard your body with well-cushioned running shoes.

- Unlike races of other distances, the marathon is a lot longer than most people's daily run—two hours plus. The ability to handle it will come after slowly building up the length of the weekly long run.

■ You'll almost certainly go through stages in the marathon when your body cries out for you to stop. Energy tends to come in waves after the 20-mile mark as glycogen levels sink. Don't despair—often a mile down the road something will change for the better.

■ You'll get dehydrated, even on a cold day. It's crucial to learn to drink water during your long training runs—and you might want to practice grabbing a drink without stopping, like most people do in a marathon to save time.

Leading into the schedules below, it will be most helpful to the runner if she has done a certain amount of base-work running prior to beginning the 12-week marathon-specific training plans. It is strongly advised that the complete beginner first visit a doctor for a checkup, then start training (*see* Chapter 1) and progress to a level of fitness at which she can run 30–40 minutes per day four times per week for three months before tackling marathon training.

Tapering
As the marathon date approaches, it is important to lighten your training load to rest the body. This is known as "tapering."

As well as cutting back on the amount of mileage you're running, be careful not to expend energy in other ways—don't clear out the garage just because you don't have a long run scheduled. Save, and store, energy! Try not to be on your feet needlessly in the week before the race.

Sharing an experience with a partner is often doubly rewarding. Why not try and hook up with another runner and aim at running the same marathon? Even if your partner isn't exactly your speed, it's possible to run parts of each other's workouts nearly every day. The shared encouragement is invaluable.

Following are three schedules—the Get-U-Round (GUR), the four-hour, and the three-hour plan. Good luck.

Training-schedule abbreviations:

Es = Easy running at a conversational pace—or at approximately 60–70 percent of your maximum heart rate.

XT = Cross-training, such as an hour of bicycling, a brisk walk, weight training, or thirty minutes of running in a swimming pool while wearing a flotation belt or vest.

F = Fartlek (Swedish for speed-play). Running with many changes of pace— slow to fast, to moderate, to sprinting, to slow again, etc.—for varying distances within a single run. An anaerobic but often-enjoyable workout.

H = Hills. The choice is yours—either run continually up and down a hill, or use a more traditional approach: sprinting up a 400-meter hill and jog down, for about ten repeats.

A = Anaerobic-threshold-pace running—approximately 15K race pace, a pace significantly faster than your marathon goal pace.

V = Interval training at VO_2 maximum, or 2-mile to 5K race pace. A speed that you feel could be maintained for not much more than 10–15 minutes.

MP = Goal marathon-pace runs.

R = Race.

Notes

■ The GUR program simply calls for running steady miles with races.

■ All types of speed running require a warmup and a cooldown. For example, F8 means a 2-mile warmup, 4 miles of fartlek, and a 2-mile cooldown. The same warmup and cooldown are included in A8.

13-Week Marathon Training Schedule

		Mon	Tue	Wed	Thu	Fri	Sat	Sun	Approx. Miles/Week
WEEK 1	GUR	*	4	*	4		*	6	14
	4-HR	A8	E5	H7	XT		E15	*	35
	3-HR	A10	E8	H8	XT		E15	6	47
	Check box	___	___	___	___		___	___	___
WEEK 2	GUR	*	6	*	5		4	10	25
	4-HR	V8	E10	XT	H7		5M R	*	30
	3-HR	V8	E12	XT	H8		10K R	E4	42
	Check box	___	___	___	___		___	___	___
WEEK 3	GUR	*	6	4	*		15	4	29
	4-HR	V8	F8	XT	E8		E18	*	44
	3-HR	V10	A10	XT	E8		E18	E4	50
	Check box	___	___	___	___		___	___	___
WEEK 4	GUR	*	7	4	*		16	4	31
	4-HR	H7	E8	A8	XT		E15	*	38
	3-HR	H8	E10	A9	XT		E16	E5	48
	Check box	___	___	___	___		___	___	___
WEEK 5	GUR	5	*	10	*		*15	4	34
	4-HR	E8	F8	XT	E10		10MR	*	39
	3-HR	E10	F10	XT	E8		½-mar R	E5	50
	Check box	___	___	___	___		___	___	___
WEEK 6	GUR	*	12	*	4		20	*	36
	4-HR	V8	E10	H7	XT		E20	*	45
	3-HR	V10	A8	E10	XT		E22	E5	55
	Check box	___	___	___	___		___	___	___

		Mon	Tue	Wed	Thu	Fri	Sat	Sun	Approx. Miles/Week
WEEK 7	GUR	*	8	*	8		*	½-mar R	32
	4-HR	A9	E15	V8	XT		E7	*	39
	3-HR	A10	E15	V8	XT		E10	E7	50
	Check box	____	____	____	____		____	____	____
WEEK 8	GUR	*	8	7	*		18	4	37
	4-HR	XT	E8	XT	F8		20M R	38	
	3-HR	XT	E10	A8	E6		20M R	E5	53
	Check box	____	____	____	____		____	____	____
WEEK 9	GUR	*	10	*	6		4	16	36
	4-HR	H7	E10	V8	XT		E15	*	40
	3-HR	H9	E10	V8	XT		MP12	E4	44
	Check box	____	____	____	____		____	____	____
WEEK 10	GUR	*	10	*	8		*	6	24
	4-HR	A8	E8	F8	XT		E20	*	44
	3-HR	A8	MP10	E8	XT		E21	E6	53
	Check box	____	____	____	____		____	____	____
WEEK 11	GUR	*	12	*	10		*	4	26
	4-HR	V8	E7	A8	XT		E16	*	39
	3-HR	V8	MP8	XT	A10		MP12	E6	44
	Check box	____	____	____	____		____	____	____
WEEK 12	GUR	*	7	*	7		*	6	20
	4-HR	V7	E6	E7	A6		E3	*	29
	3-HR	V8	E8	MP5	E4		E5	5K R	36
	Check box	____	____	____	____		____	____	____
WEEK 13	GUR	*	4	*	2		2	*	MARATHON
	4-HR	E4	E3	E3	*		E3	*	MARATHON
	3-HR	E4	E4	E3	*		E3	*	MARATHON
	Check box	____	____	____	____		____	____	____

Time Predictor for the Marathon

If this is your first marathon race, the table below may help you decide on your pace. Simply find a time that you've recently run at one of the standard shorter distances, and follow the line across to find the indicated marathon time.

5Km	10Km	½-mar	marathon
15:00	32:00	1:10	2:30
16:00	34:00	1:15	2:40
17:00	36:00	1:20	2:50
18:00	38:00	1:25	3:00
19:00	40:00	1:30	3:10
20:00	42:00	1:35	3:30
21:00	44:00	1:40	3:40
23:00	48:00	1:50	4:00
26:00	54:00	2:05	4:30
30:00	1:08	2:28	5:30

Training Commitment

Although sitting at home and watching the elite athletes glide over the roads can give you the impression that running is a God-given talent, even the swift of foot sweat. The smooth cadence and apparent ease of effort comes from practicing day after day, year after year. At an elite level, marathon training is far from easy. It is demanding and time-consuming. Jerry Lawson, the former American record-holder at 25K and the marathon, posted weeks of more than 200 miles of running in preparation for some of his races.

1999's male champion, Joseph Chebet of Kenya, trained for five months with the sole goal of being victorious in New York. "I lived for this race. I did nothing but train, eat, and sleep for New York," he says.

Juma Ikangaa, the Tanzanian national record-holder, used to run as far as he could at marathon race pace out on the roads of Arusha, his hometown. "I would often collapse and need a vehicle to take me home," he remembers. Gidamis Shahanga, who clocked an impressive 48:06 for the first ten miles in New York in 1983 before fading to sixth, had heard that New York's was a very hilly course: "I trained on the hills for up to three hours at a time before coming to New York. I found the course rather flat."

HOW A CHAMPION TRAINS

A week of training from Douglas Wakiihuri, the 1992 NYC Marathon winner. Douglas typically trained twice each day!

Sunday:	Long run, 45–50k, steady pace
Monday:	A.M. Easy recovery run, 1 hour
	P.M. Easy recovery run, 45 minutes
Tuesday:	A.M. Intervals: 15 × 1000 meters at marathon race pace
	P.M. Easy recovery run, 1½ hours
Wednesday:	A.M. Long run: 1½ hours
Thursday:	A.M. Hill repeats, 1 hour
	P.M. Easy recovery run, 45 minutes
Friday:	A.M. Tempo run, 12K at marathon pace
	P.M. 1 hour steady
Saturday:	A.M. 1 hour steady
	P.M. 1 hour steady

Great Britain's Ron Hill, a European and Commonwealth Champion and one of the first runners under the 2:10 barrier, has this piece of advice on how to train for a marathon: "It was just a matter of a lot of hard training."

Moses Tanui learned about the marathon the hard way in New York in 1993: "I had the world record in the half-marathon [59:47] and had taken the silver in the world track championships [at 10,000 meters]. I thought I was ready, but I had not done enough long runs, and I faded badly. I had not learned about marathon running." Tanui, after leading early, finished in a disappointing tenth place with a 2:15:36. After "learning," Tanui improved his personal record to 2:06:16, then the third-fastest time in history.

Kim Jones, runner-up in the 1989 NYC Marathon, has a treadmill in her home. Thus, if the weather becomes too treacherous for fast running, she has no excuse not to log a quality session.

2000 Boston Marathon winner Elijah Lagat recalls, "I would run at night for hours to try and get in shape. I knew success would come if I did the hard work. It did, but it took a number of years."

RACE-DAY TIPS

■ Buy a subway token to get to the marathon transportation buses. This way you don't have to take change and risk losing a loose coin, or find that your subway card is expired.

■ Dress in layers of old clothes that you can discard.

■ Pack warm clothes in your baggage to be transported to the finishing line.

■ Unless it's quite warm out, take an old, loose-fitting T-shirt and cut out a "TV screen" hole to display your bib number. Wear it for the first few miles until you've warmed up, then discard it.

■ Take a bottle of water, toilet paper, petroleum jelly, and gloves with you to the starting area.

■ During the race, try to avoid water getting on your feet from drink-station spillage or puddles.

■ Try to find a rhythm in the early miles.

■ Plan your hydration, for before and during the race.

■ Stick with your plan. A rational, well-thought-out plan always beats a last-minute miracle marathon plan.

■ Try to relax.

Tegla Loroupe calls hill running the reason for her two NYC titles. "I do a lot of hill work for the marathon. This makes you very strong, and you are able to push in the park."

Hugh Jones, third in the 1981 race, says, "I would do a session where I would run five-K in fifteen minutes, then relax [!] with a sixteen-minute five-K, continue straight into another fifteen-minute five-K, and finish with one more sixteen-minute five-K run." When you can duplicate this session, you're ready to challenge the best at New York!

Marathon Training Diet

It's important to eat properly while training for a marathon. A balanced diet is far better than any fad diet. Try to include plenty of carbohydrates, an adequate amount of protein, and a smaller amount of fat. Generally speaking, an equation of 60 percent carbohydrate, 25 percent protein, and 15 percent fat has long been considered a healthy marathoner's diet. In my years of training and eating with world-class marathoners, I've found the equation to be more like 70 percent carbohydrates, 18 percent protein, and 12 percent fat.

A major consideration is that you must increase your caloric intake to give your body the energy to run. We always have virtually unlimited choices at the dinner table, and making healthy ones will help your training. (For instance, to cut down on fats, you might choose mustard over mayonnaise and jelly over butter.) The little things will combine to make a big difference.

A golden rule is to drink, drink, and then drink some more water! Water is the body's motor oil: It allows the joints and muscles to operate smoothly. Water acts as the body's coolant, helps with digestion, and transports nutrients to the cells as well as fuel to the muscles. You should never reach a state of thirst during any part of the day.

It's a mistake to think that you can simply drink a little extra in the last day or two before a race and come to the starting line well hydrated. You should begin to take in extra water *when you begin your marathon training*, and during your long runs, try to drink every three or four miles along the route.

A good test is the color of your urine—it should be clear, or nearly so.

The need for water increases with the temperature and humidity. Water is the main ingredient of sweat, so the more you're sweating, the more you should be drinking—before, during, and after your runs.

If your diet is balanced, taking supplements is unnecessary. In Tanzania, most of the country's best athletes live in the village of Arusha. It is here that former NYC course record-holder Juma Ikangaa grew up. In the local "pharmacist's shop," the only supplements available were vitamin C tablets. Did Juma grow up eating them? No.

The same conditions prevail in Kenya and Ethiopia. Don't be fooled into thinking that the world's best runners are supplement-takers. It's as far from the truth as you can get!

Nutrition for Optimum Sports Performance

Nutritional needs differ from person to person, depending on such factors as age, lifestyle, body mass, and metabolism. However, there are some building blocks that remain universal, the key word being *balance*.

It's better to think not so much of "good foods" and "bad foods," but rather of good and bad diets. Being a runner does not demand a major change from any balanced diet.

As you burn more calories with exercise, your caloric needs will increase. You must eat more food than a sedentary person does, and you'll be able to do so without gaining weight.

A balanced diet with a wide variety of foods is best; this lessens the chances of any nutritional deficiency. It's important to eat a combination of all the major food types.

All the Essential Nutrients are Contained in the Foods That Make Up a Balanced Diet

- Carbohydrate

- Protein

- Fat

- Minerals

- Fiber (not a nutrient, but necessary)

- Water (not a nutrient, but essential)

A point of interest: Alcohol is a nutrient—but not necessary.

A diet for the athlete must provide an adequate supply of energy and nutrients to meet the demands not only of training, but also of recovery after exercise, when, for instance, the muscles rebuild themselves stronger than they were before the last workout.

As with most things in life, a lack of education or knowledge can lead to disastrous results. The sports-nutrition business is huge and ever-growing; seemingly every day a new wonder drug appears on the scene with promises that it will aid performance.

In September 2000, the International Amateur Athletic Federation's top twenty ranked male distance runners were *all* African-born, and the majority of them were East African. To find a simple aspirin tablet in this part of the world can be a challenge, let alone the latest oxygen-boosting, cell-building wonder pill. It's quite clear that most of the people who win international marathons do so by virtue of years of hard training and sound natural diets.

Insufficient knowledge about foods and nutrition is often the path to poor eating habits. Train hard, and try not to neglect your nutritional needs.

Natural-based diets are the key to a winning formula. There are many sports nutrition companies on the scene, but very few offer products without refined ingredients and added chemicals. The Leppin Sports company of Great Britain is one manufacturer that has made a product that uses natural foods with no additives. "Many runners are now using our "squeezy" [an energy gel package] for marathon running. It is pure carbohydrate, with no stimulants (caffeine for example) that can upset the stomach during running," says Ivar Trausti of Leppin. Likewise, the Leppin carbo-loading drink is almost pure carbs—the most per ounce that I could find on the market. This is a refreshing break in a field that has long been tainted by substitute "miracle" ingredients that subtract from the real ethics of running: hard work and a good natural diet.

Elite Marathon Runners' Favorite Foods:

Dionicio Ceron, three-time winner of the London Marathon:

"Chicken, rice, beans . . . the food of Mexico."

Lornah Kiplagat, 2:22 marathoner and two-time winner of the Los Angeles Marathon:

"Ugali and vegetables." Ugali is a stiff porridge made in Kenya from the flour of ground maize.

Eddy Hellebuyck, 2:11 U.S. marathoner:

"My wife Shawn's home cooking." [Shawn often cooks pasta, with spinach and other fresh vegetables, for the family meals.]

Andres Espinosa, 1993 New York Champion:

"Mexican food: I love beans and rice."

Catherina McKiernan, 2:22 marathoner, winner of the Berlin, Amsterdam, and London marathons:

"Meat and potatoes."

The demands of marathon running will help to tune you in to a better diet if you pay attention as your body asks for good food to fuel its efforts.

It is paramount to remember that although diet alone will not guarantee success, an insufficient diet will limit the athlete's ability to achieve his best, and may also increase the chance of injury.

Q-and-A for the Marathoner

Q: *How much extra energy do I need for running?*
A: Each mile burns approximately 100 calories.

Q: *Is it just carbohydrates that I need for training?*
A: A balance of carbohydrate, protein, and fat is needed, but carbs should make up more than half of the calorie intake.

Q: *How much protein do athletes need?*
A: Protein needs are still under debate. According to one NYC sports nutritionist, we don't need as much as we are led to believe. Again, if we look at the diets of the champion African athletes, the main source of protein is usually a bowl of beans and a glass of milk per day: great quality, but not much quantity.

Q: *How much fat should be in an athlete's diet?*
A: A small amount, and you should aim for the right kinds of fat. Steer clear of saturated and hydrogenated fats. Olive oil and nuts are excellent fat sources. Even the skinniest body has enough fat energy stored to run two consecutive marathons!

Q: *Are vitamin and mineral supplements necessary in the athlete's diet?*

A: Only if the diet is poor. If you're eating a well-balanced diet of natural foods, they aren't necessary.

Q: *What are the extra fluid requirements during marathon training?*

A: Try to drink a glass of water for every hour you're awake, plus an extra 32-ounce bottle for post-training. And that's for *cool-weather* training.

Q: *What is the best way to recover, using nutrition, after a workout?*

A: Nutritionists seem to agree that a combination of carbohydrate and protein within thirty minutes after a workout promotes optimum recovery. Thus a tuna sandwich would be ideal.

Q: *Should I change my diet before a race?*

A: Yes; below we'll look at the concept of carbohydrate loading. Also, staying away from high-fiber foods and lactose products often helps athletes avoid stomach problems during a race. The stomach is in a state of jitters before a race, and it's a good idea to eat easily digestable plain foods, such as oatmeal, rice, and toast. Fats are notoriously slow to digest and are not recommended.

Q: *What about special needs for a vegetarian runner?*

A: If a vegetarian runner is eating a wholesome diet, there should be no need for worry. William Tanui won an Olympic gold medal at 800 meters and has never eaten meat; Mark Yatich won the prestigious Falmouth Road Race and has eaten meat only a handful of times in his entire life.

Q: *Are there special requirements for female runners?*

A: The female athlete should take care to maintain proper iron levels and make sure to eat some extra calcium. Otherwise, the diet for men and women is the same.

These are simply guidelines, and should be taken as such.

Carbohydrate loading

The better your diet, the better your chances of standing up to the rigors of marathon running. Carbohydrates are "burned" in muscle tissue as fuel during exercise. Good carbohydrate sources include pasta, rice, and potatoes.

CHANGING TIMES

In 1970, Gary Muhrcke won the inaugural NYC Marathon, recording a time of 2:31:38. Thirteen years later, as a 43-year-old, Muhrcke ran the marathon again, in the faster time of 2:31:00—but this result gave him 197th place!

The top African runners have a diet as high as 85 percent carbohydrate. Take, for example, Tegla Loroupe, the 1994 and 1995 NYC Marathon champion:

Breakfast	Two cups of hot sweet milky tea, two slices of bread with jelly
Midmorning	More tea
Lunch	Spaghetti with a tomato-based sauce
Dinner	Ugali*, green vegetables, tomatoes, and a little beef

No matter which country's runners you ask, top marathoners will tell you that they stock up on carbohydrates for the energy to go the distance. Gelindo Bordin, Italy's 1988 Olympic marathon champion, was asked at the post-race banquet for his "training secrets." He smiled and replied, "Pasta."

---

*Ugali, the Kenyan food staple—a thick porridge made from maize meal and water—is said to be one of the purest forms of complex carbohydrate.

The Last Few Days Diet

Starting on the Wednesday prior to a Sunday race, begin to increase the proportion (of carbohydrates) in your diet, and commensurately reduce the proportions of protein and fat.

On Friday night, a good meal might be pasta with marinara sauce and chicken. A good suggestion is to eat the exact same meal on Saturday night if it's caused no problems the first time. You'll forgo the worry of a bad stomach reaction.

Here's an example of a daily diet providing 500 grams of carbohydrates—ideal for stocking the body's supplies for the demands of running a marathon. The total caloric value is 3,000 calories per day.

Breakfast	Large bowl of oatmeal (70g)
	Glass of low-fat milk
	Jam or fruit
	2 slices of bread, small amount of margarine, 30g cheese, and 15g hamburger
	Glass of orange juice
Lunch	100g roast chicken
	Large portion cooked rice (100g uncooked) with vegetable sauce
	Vegetable salad
Dinner	Spaghetti (140g uncooked) with meat sauce
	Vegetable salad
	Bread roll
	Cooked apple with ice cream
Supper	Bowl of cereal
	Glass of low-fat milk
	Bagel
	Banana or orange

The Pasta Party at Tavern on the Green

Included in each NYC Marathon entrant's goody bag is a ticket for the Pasta Party the day before the race. This event begins at 3 P.M. at the Tavern on the Green restaurant, meters away from the finish line in Central Park. Runners get the chance to eat plenty of pasta in a buffet format. The site of Tavern on the Green used to be a holding pen for sheep that grazed in a nearby meadow. Nowadays it's the location of a top-class restaurant known for its beautiful and unusual surroundings.

The pros of the event are a free meal shared with a horde of enthusiastic and excited fellow runners. However, partygoers can end up standing on their feet too long, chatting late into the night, and overeating. Keep the plate-count down to two. Carbohydrate loading isn't an excuse to stuff yourself with as much food as you can! You want to wake up the next day with no stomach discomfort.

A fireworks display is held in conjunction with the Pasta Party at 7:30 P.M.

If you're traveling to New York, remember to check that your favorite foods will be available. If you're staying at a hotel, call ahead of your arrival and ask what's available. Be prepared: If you must, travel with dry ingredients and make your own pre-race breakfast. Before the 1998 Berlin Marathon, hotel guests looked on in awe at the elite athletes as they shoveled down plates of spaghetti at six o'clock in the morning!

Chapter Five

Where to Stay and Orientation

What to Do When You First Arrive in the City

Welcome to New York! First things first—once you arrive in the city, you should take a moment to get your bearings.

Information Center: Go to pick up brochures, maps, and coupons for discounts and special deals. The center has a multilingual staff on hand to help and to advise you on how best to enjoy your stay in New York City. Tickets can also be purchased from here to many of the city's attractions.

Orientation in Manhattan

Think of Manhattan as a chessboard. There is a grid system of named or numbered avenues that run north and south on the island, and numbered streets that run east and west. Down in Greenwich Village there is no system, and getting lost is commonplace, even for locals. Above Washington Square, the East Side and the West Side are divided by Fifth Avenue. Cross-street address numbers begin at Fifth Avenue and usually grow in increments of 100 per block as one travels either east (toward the East River) or west (toward the Hudson River).

Tourists often get lost only because they are not sure whether they are headed east or west. A useful tip is to look at the traffic: The even-numbered streets are almost always one-way heading east, and the odd-numbered head west.

Airports

There are three major airports serving the New York area:

John F. Kennedy International (JFK) is in Queens, 15 miles (24 km) from the center of Manhattan

Fiorello La Guardia International (LGA) is also in Queens, 8 miles (13 km) east of Manhattan

Newark International (EWR) is in New Jersey, 10 miles (16 km) west of Manhattan

JFK has a fixed-price taxi service (currently 30 dollars) operating to the city. Busses run to the center of Manhattan for 14 dollars. From La Guardia and JFK, one of the best bargains in the city is a free bus that drops you at the subway station, from which a dollar-fifty ride takes you wherever you want to go on the subway.

SOME NEW YORK CITY FACTS:

Population 7,500,000
Area 300 square miles (780 square km)
Elevation 87 feet (27 m)
State New York
Time Zone Eastern (GMT minus five hours)
Telephone area codes
Manhattan: 212, 646, and 917
Other boroughs: 718, 347, and 917

The Districts of Manhattan at a Glance

Downtown Manhattan
Financial District
Includes the South Street Seaport, Wall Street, the New York Stock Exchange, and Battery Park City.

Chinatown
The largest Chinatown in the United States. Packed with inexpensive restaurants and gadget stores.

SoHo
Quaint small streets and fine galleries.

Little Italy
The best Italian restaurants and cafés.

Lower East Side
A colorful residential area with many immigrant-group enclaves.

Greenwich Village
Centered around Washington Square Park and New York University, the famous bohemian capital still boasts great music clubs, pubs, and theaters.

East Village
Known for the punk and far-out side of town. Tattoo and body-piercing parlors are the norm.

TriBeCa
It stands for "Triangle below Canal" and is home to many galleries, fine restaurants, and artists' lofts. A trendy and expensive area.

Gramercy Park (18th to 21st Streets between Park Avenue South and Third Avenue)
An old, upscale residential area amidst the inner-city bustle.

Chelsea (between 14th and 30th Streets, west of Park Avenue)
Clothing stores galore. Includes the Flatiron district.

Midtown Manhattan

A clamorous and clangorous part of town. Definitely in the heart of the city, and with the feeling that you're close to everything. Many of the larger hotels are located here.

Midtown West Side

Famous for Broadway, the theater district, the garment district, and Times Square.

Midtown East Side

Home to Carnegie Hall, the Museum of Modern Art (MOMA), the Empire State Building, Radio City Music Hall, St. Patrick's Cathedral, Rockefeller Center (and skating rink), and Grand Central Terminal.

Uptown Manhattan

Central Park

The jewel of the city, and not only for the runner. A zoo, the Metropolitan Museum of Art, Shakespeare in the Park, outdoor concerts, and *much* more.

Upper West Side

Beautiful residential areas, homes to the famous. Known for artists, intellectuals, and streetside restaurants. Includes Lincoln Center, Columbia University, the Museum of Natural History, and the huge Cathedral of St. John the Divine. For many, *the* place to live in Manhattan, and housing prices reflect this trend.

Upper East Side

The wealthiest neighborhood on earth (really!) includes Museum Mile (with its numerous museums, most prominently the Met), Gracie Mansion, and Madison Avenue, probably the most expensive shopping center in the world. The Upper East Side is recommended for its serenity within the city.

Harlem

The historic African-American and Hispanic neighborhood. Those who know the area will check out the famous Apollo Theatre.

Inwood and Washington Heights

Worth a visit for the Cloisters, the Dyckman Farmhouse, and Audubon Terrace.

A NEIGHBORHOOD OF CELEBRITIES

The Upper East Side is probably home to more famous people per square mile than any other neighborhood in the world. (Even Hollywood, because people aren't so densely packed there!) During the marathon's 16th through 18th miles, you'll be very close to many of their homes. Don't get too distracted!

As you run up First Avenue, you'll pass 61st Street, where talk-show host Joan Rivers has a town house. Neil Diamond has an apartment on 63rd Street close to the park. Kitty Carlisle is on 64th, and both Elle McPherson and Al Pacino are on 68th. Sidney Poitier has an address on 70th Street. On First Avenue, the runners pass the Silver Spoon Café between 70th and 71st; it was here that Fred Lebow would come for his morning bowl of oatmeal. Fred lived around the corner on 72nd Street, where Frank Sinatra had a New York apartment. On 73rd near Fifth Avenue is Woody Allen's house. Lena Horne has a place on 74th. As the route passes 76th Street, you can see Sammy Davis, Jr.'s old building on the left. The mayor of New York, Mike Bloomberg, lives on 79th; on 80th Imelda Marcos used to stay in a six-story mansion. Jackie Onassis lived on 84th, near the park; Walter Cronkite still does. Isabella Rossellini owns a pink town house on 85th Street. Mary Tyler Moore's apartment is on 86th, down near the East River. The route passes the mayoral offices, Gracie Mansion, at 88th. Billy Joel lived on 90th in a walk-up between First and Second Avenues before his success with his album *The Stranger,* Anthony Quinn had an apartment across First. Up into Harlem, the route passes 127th Street, where the writer Langston Hughes lived, and Marcus Garvey Park, which honors the 1920s.

In the final mile, the race passes the famous Plaza Hotel. Films such as *Home Alone* and *Crocodile Dundee* have been filmed at this location.

New York Yankee Mickey Mantle lived at the Ritz Carlton Hotel on Central Park

South. The hotel is now being turned into apartments, but Mantle's restaurant is still close by.

As you make the turn at Columbus Circle, glance up at the Trump building, where author Robin Cook owns the penthouse apartment. Although the course now runs into the park, adjacent to the finishing stretch is 64th Street, where Madonna has an apartment on the fifth floor of Number 1.

Hotels

Here are ten top hotels, listed alphabetically, with locations close to Central Park and the majority of New York's attractions.

New York accommodation is rather expensive, and on the marathon week it's also rather hectic. It pays to plan in advance, and make an early booking if you intend to stay at a hotel.

Belvedere*
319 West 48th Street
(212) 245-7000
$190 single/double

A first-class Baroque-styled hotel in the historic theater district. Entertainment center with pay-per-view movies, Web TV, and Nintendo. Custom kitchenettes with microwave, refrigerator, and coffeemaker. Individual climate control unit. Modem-ready telephones with voice mail. Personal safe. Full-size iron and ironing board.

Shower massage. Hair dryer. Gilchrist & Soames designer bath amenities. Within walking distance of Central Park!

Chelsea
222 West 23rd Street
(212) 243-3700
$100 single/double

*Two-night minimum required

A legendary NYC hotel with a who's who of guests. Why not ask for the very room Madonna lived in when she was a struggling artist? A five-minute subway ride to Central Park, and very close to the running trail along the West Side Highway. Cheaper shared accommodation available. The dormitory rooms include linens and feature sitting-room areas. The private rooms can accommodate from one to four people.

Clarion*
3 East 40th Street
(212) 532-4860
$229 single/double
Health club available

"Best value on Fifth Avenue—a fashionable address with affordable rates." Built in 1990, the Clarion has more than 180 guest rooms featuring either a queen-sized bed or one or two double beds; two telephones, each with two lines and one with speakerphone; voice mail; 25" TV with complimentary cable service; express checkout; daily newspaper; in-room coffeemakers; iron and ironing board; well-lit work area; waffle-weave bathrobes, imported Egyptian cotton towels, hair dryers; waffle-weave triple-sheeted beds; Bath & Body Works bathroom products; bottled water upon arrival; umbrellas; task lighting and easy-access electrical outlets. Rooms with queen-size beds also feature a sitting area with either sofa bed or a lounge chair with ottoman.

Empire**
44 West 63rd Street
(212) 265-7400
$195/single
$215 double/twins

*Two-night minimum required
**Three-night minimum required

$240 queen/double-double

$255 mini-suite

$285 junior suite

Full health club facilities, one block from Central Park. "Best kept secret on the West Side." Offers an elegant, European style perfect for both leisure and business travelers. With Central Park steps away and Lincoln Center right next door, the Empire is ideally suited for guests seeking a West Side experience only minutes from bustling Midtown and vibrant Times Square. The West Side has a tempo all its own with some of the best dining, shopping, entertainment, and cultural events that New York has to offer.

Essex House

160 Central Park South

(212) 247-0300

$335 city view

$350 park view

Health and beauty spa, running maps of Central Park. Magnificently restored to its original art deco beauty, Essex House is a sublime oasis of elegance and style in the heart of midtown Manhattan. Very close to Carnegie Hall, Fifth Avenue shopping, and the Museum of Modern Art. The hotel's dedicated staff attends to guests in 20[!] languages, and a full-service business center offers everything from secretarial support to private offices for rent. Relax with a spa pedicure, body treatment, or massage. Next door to Central Park.

Fitzpatrick Grand Central*

141 East 44th Street

(212) 355-0100

$205 single/double

*Two-night minimum required

Offers a full array of deluxe amenities and services with warm Irish hospitality. Complimentary access to a health-and-fitness club located just a few blocks away.

InterContinental*
111 East 48th Street
(212) 755-5900
(800) 327-0200
$269 single/double

A short jog from Central Park. Extensive gym (fitness center with circuit training, Lifecycles, treadmills, StairMaster), pool, sauna, steamroom, and massage—and furthermore, the fitness manager is a 2:48 marathoner. Located just off Park Avenue in the center of Manhattan. Close to midtown business, fashionable shops, restaurants, museums, and Broadway. 682 guest rooms. Barclay Bar and Grill with entertainment nightly. Laundry and valet, voice mail, two-line phones with data jack, TV with cable forecasts, in-room video checkout, concierge, shops, business center. This hotel complies with the Americans with Disabilities Act.

Mayflower**
15 Central Park West
(212) 265-0060
$225 single
$245 double
$320 one-bedroom suite

Small gym, but a stone's throw from the park. The Mayflower is perfectly situated within the vibrant culture of the Upper West Side and overlooks Central Park from 61st Street. Intimate European charm and ambiance. The best of Manhattan is only steps away!

*Two-night minimum required
**Three-night minimum required

The guest rooms and suites provide a haven of comfort and tranquility for business and leisure visitors. With its marvelous location and gracious service, this is an excellent choice from which to begin your New York experience.

Trump International

1 Central Park West (at 59th Street)

(212) 299-1000

$250–$350

Opened January 1997. Its location makes for an ideal Manhattan base. Luxurious yet functional, with a great gym. Floor-to-ceiling windows offer spectacular views of Central Park and the Manhattan skyline.

Warwick*

65 West 54th Street

(212) 247-2700

$275 single/double

The Warwick is mere steps from Broadway's bright lights, Central Park, Carnegie Hall, Rockefeller Center, Fifth Avenue, the Museum of Modern Art, and countless dining and shopping opportunities. Carey Grant lived here for twelve years, and it was also the NYC hotel choice of the Beatles.

For cheaper alternatives:

Boulevard Motor Inn, Queens (718) 457-1400

Days Hotel (800) 572-6232

Habitat Hotel (800) 497-6028

*Two-night minimum required

Holiday Inn, Soho (212) 966-8898

Holiday Inn, Midtown (212) 581-8100

Madison Hotel (800) 9-MADISON

Novotel (800) NOVOTEL

Cheaper still, try the YMCA. The Y's not only have amazing fitness centers but are hubs for travelers who want the heart and beat of the city without the NYC price. Book early!

Vanderbilt Y, 224 East 47th Street, (212) 756-9600

West Side Y, 5 West 63rd Street, (212) 875-4100

Harlem Y, 180 West 135th Street, (212) 281-4100

Another option is to rent a furnished apartment. Call Urban Ventures at (212) 594-5650. Examples: One bedroom in west midtown that sleeps four (assuming everyone is friendly) for $150 a night; two bedrooms, two baths in west midtown for $240.

These websites offer a great guide to a wide variety of city hotels.

www.123-newyorkhotels.com

www.newyork.com/hotels

www.hotels-ny.com

www.allny.com

and in the higher range,

www.luxuryhotels-ny.com

14 TIPS FOR SURVIVING IN NEW YORK CITY

- The best place to hail a taxi in NYC is near a luxury hotel.

- Before stepping into a city cab, check that the driver understands your language and recognizes your destination.

- The NY "attitude" was created by tourists who ask directions of New Yorkers who are late for work. Ask someone who looks like she has time to spare.

- A major New York scam: While shopping for bargains on electronic products watch out for refurbished and repackaged second-hand goods.

- Problems while shopping? Department of Consumer Affairs telephone number: (212) 487-4398.

- Don't stop on the sidewalk if someone asks you for a match; keep walking.

- Walk toward the curb side of the street, not near the alleyways or doorways.

- Don't expose large amounts of cash or other wealth.

- Never keep your wallet in an outer pocket.

- Never leave your handbag on the empty seat next to you or on the back of your seat—these are invitations for its removal. Pickpockets strike every seven minutes, on average, in the United States.

- If you are claustrophobic: Simply put, avoid the NYC subway at rush hour!

- Rest rooms are often hard to find when you need them. Most savvy New Yorkers simply march through a restaurant with an air that says they have a table. Hotels are a good bet, though the restrooms are often hidden behind the concierge's desk or on the second floor.

■ If you have rented or borrowed a car and it has disappeared, after calling the police also call (212) TOW-AWAY.

■ New York is the king of cities. Whatever happens there happens with gusto. It is not a dangerous city, especially per capita, but be prepared for encountering the good and the bad.

Where to Run in NYC

Manhattan
West Side
On the West Side of Manhattan, near the Hudson River, is an ideal running route for the marathoner: A traffic-free, completely flat path with scenic waterfront views is fast becoming a Mecca for runners.

A tour along the West Side promenade that runs from the George Washington Bridge to Battery Park makes this route ideal for runners staying on the west side of the city. The path, recently surfaced with tarmac, is flat and ideal for those easy pre-marathon runs. Access to the path is available at a number of points:

Transport: To reach the southernmost tip of the run, take the N or R train to the Bowling Green subway stop. For the northernmost point, take the A train to 181st Street. The path is accessible at many points between these two—from almost anywhere, just head west. Between Chambers Street and 68th Street, there are pedestrian cross-walks across the West Side Highway at regular intervals.

ACCESS:

By subway: A, C, or E train to 14th Street or Battery Park City

By bus: #14 to West Street (between West 15th and 18th street) or #9 + #20 to Battery Park City.

By taxi: Ask for 14th Street and West Street.

By car: The Port Authority garage is just off the West Side Highway at West 15th Street.

For a six-mile out-and-back run, cross the West Side Highway at West 14th Street and run south for the more picturesque route. Follow the path and keep the water on your right. The Statue of Liberty can be seen to your right, and after a couple of miles you'll pass the financial district of New York on your left. Turn around at the southern tip of Battery Park after three miles and run back uptown to your starting point. Public bathrooms are available at Chelsea Piers on West 23rd Street, and there are many restaurants in the financial area that can be used for water and bathroom stops.

For fewer miles, simply double back sooner.

Although the path runs a full twelve miles, there are certain points where, at this writing, construction of the path is not yet complete. During marathon week, it's always advisable to keep training distances at a minimum, and it's worthwhile to take public transport to the clear path rather than chance any of the iffy areas. It's a good idea to stay within the stretch between 59th Street and Battery Park.

Central Park

There is simply no better place to run in Manhattan, period. Each day, thousands of runners flock to this urban oasis to enjoy the best greenery in one of the world's greatest cities. There is choice aplenty, including a variety of running surfaces, and the chance to avoid the traffic.

The main entrance to the six-mile road loop is at the Engineers' Gate at 90th Street and Fifth Avenue. In the Fred Lebow era, all NYRR races began at this point; ever-swelling numbers have caused race organizers to relocate.

THE SIX-MILE LOOP: There are two inner recreation lanes—one for bicycles and the innermost for runners. Runners should run counterclockwise in the recreation lane to the left. Cars are not permitted in either of these two lanes. The full road loop is a smidgen over six miles. Simply run without making any turns and the road will lead you over a variety of hills and back to your starting point.

There are three easy modifications of this basic loop.

The four-mile loop: Follow the six-mile loop, but at 102nd Street (approximately ¾ mile north of 90th Street) turn left at the first major intersection. The transverse road is 400 meters long; at the end, take another left. You're now running south on the west side of the park. Continue on the main road until you arrive at the 72nd Street transverse (approximately another 1½ miles). At the traffic light, turn left and run back across to the east side. (As you cross, to your left will be the famous Bethesda Fountain.) At the end of the transverse (approximately ¼ mile), bear left, run downhill past the Boathouse restaurant, and continue up a steep hill. This road will lead you back to your starting point.

The five-mile upper loop: This includes the notorious Northern Hill, perhaps the toughest climb in Central Park. Follow the directions for the four-mile loop, but do not take the first left turn; instead, follow the road down past the Lasker open-air swimming pool. Once you've climbed the Northern Hill—a steep 600 meters—you'll be on the West Side, and you can resume the four-mile-loop directions.

The five-mile lower loop: Follow the directions for the four-mile loop until you arrive at the 72nd Street transverse. Instead of taking the left, continue straight and follow the road around the southern end of the park.

THE RESERVOIR Perhaps the most traveled running path in the world. This loop around the reservoir is exactly 1.577 miles, and it's marked every 20 yards. From the Engineers' Gate at East 90th Street, walk up the stone stairs and onto the cinder path. Run counterclockwise and enjoy the terrific views of Manhattan. The completely flat path makes this an ideal pre-marathon loop—and there's no chance to get lost, either. The surface of the reservoir is specially designed to dissipate water, so large puddles are unusual. There is a slight camber to help the drainage, and the surface is a fine-grain cinder gravel. The upkeep of this running path is costly, and the NYRR donates large sums of money to help with it.

THE BRIDLE PATH   Just below the reservoir is a rough dirt track that runs in a 1.66-mile loop. Be careful, as it's called "the bridle path" for a reason: Horses are indeed ridden on it. The terrain can be muddy after a rain. A 2.5-mile and a 5-mile extension of this loop can be made by making a right hairpin turn one-third of a mile north of East 90th Street and following a gravel/dirt path. However, for first-timers in the park, the risk of getting lost makes this option less wise.

THE GREAT LAWN   This large field allows the runner to stay on the grass. The lawn is situated in the middle of the park between 80th and 85th streets, both East and West. Keep to the perimeter of the grass for a 600-meter loop—or run on the concrete path that circles the oval lawn.

The Park's Amenities   There are many water fountains and seventeen public bathrooms throughout the park. Four water fountains can be found at the park's East 90th Street entrance, and many others dot the road loop around the park and can easily be spotted by runners. The fountains are turned off from December to March.

Public bathrooms can be found at the boathouse, at the tennis courts, at the children's playground, at the southern end of the park, along the 72nd Street transverse, and at the Conservatory Gardens, to name a few. There are information posts at the park entrance that give full details of the whereabouts of the park's amenities.

ACCESS:

  By subway: 1 train to 59th Street.

                   4, 5, or 6 trains: all stations between 59th and 110th streets.

                   A and C trains: 59th to 110th streets.

                   N or R train: to 59th Street.

On weekdays, the park is closed to vehicle traffic between 10 A.M. and 3 P.M. and between 7 P.M. and 10 P.M. On weekends, no traffic is permitted from 7 P.M. Friday to 6 A.M. Monday. Be warned, however: On weekdays, cars will drive through the park from the 5th Avenue entrance to East 72nd Street, throughout the day. Emergency vehicles also use the park, and vehicles belonging to the parks department use the roads regularly. Caution is advised at all times.

> "When I first moved to New Jersey, I tried running everywhere. The lower parts of Manhattan, the North Jersey shoreline, and most other places. But now I just take the train and run in Central Park. It's easily the best place."
>
> —Kiet Vo, New Jersey runner

Lower East Side Pedestrian Pathways

Far harder to get to than its western counterpart, the Lower East Side's riverside route does lead past one of Manhattan's few open all-weather running tracks. A run along the East River can extend as far south as Battery Park and as far north as 34th Street, primarily right on the waterfront on paved paths. The total distance one-way is approximately four miles.

The Tartan-surfaced running track, located across the Roosevelt Drive from the eastern end of 6th Street (and visible from the riverside path), has public rest rooms and changing facilities that are open between 8 A.M. and 3 P.M.

ACCESS:

    By subway: 6 train to 33rd Street.

The route is traffic free, and it's less populated than the West Side pedestrian path. However, the area is less pleasing to the eye than the West Side, the Fulton Fish Market along the route has olfactory drawbacks and the water fountains and bathrooms are scarce.

Upper West Side

Skirting the Hudson River on the west side of Manhattan are 350 acres of prime parkland ideally suited for running. It is possible to run along the entire west side of Manhattan, but a particularly agreeable stretch is through Riverside Park.

The most popular section to run is from 72nd Street up to 110th Street, where the runner gets a choice of continuing either along the flat, traffic-free path by the water's edge, or through the park itself—a mere 100 yards inland. The only drawback of this second option is that occasionally the route includes some long flights of stairs leading up to and down from Riverside Drive; these might be a bit arduous for the marathoner running easy in the few days before the race. Several cafés along the route can serve as drink and/or bathroom stops, and there are plenty of portable toilets in the park, too. There are five yellow emergency telephones by the playgrounds between 76th and 105th streets.

Sample Upper West Side Run   Start at the statue of Eleanor Roosevelt at the 72nd Street entrance to the park. (Local runner Tom Hayes says that plenty of training partners can be found at this spot each morning willing to guide the newcomer around the park.) Bear left down the hill, go through the underpass, and proceed down to the water's edge. Then run north, with the water on your left. After a mile and a half the path splits; take the right turn, which will take you under the 96th Street underpass. Do your hill work up to the flat promenade. Run along this for another half-mile, at which point you'll again have a choice of routes. Avoid the dirt trail and take the tarmac path for a further half mile. Turn around and run back to finish five miles.

At the turnaround point, there is a stairway leading up to the Riverside Church. You can climb these stairs and continue north if you're looking for a longer run. For those wanting to add some speedwork to the run, there's a 200-meter cinder track at the southern end of the path by the Hudson River, and at 101st Street there's an asphalt track around a soccer field.

The promenades are shared by dog-walkers, skaters, and cyclists; run with caution.

ACCESS:
> **By subway:**   1, 2, 3, or 9 train to 72nd Street.

Upper East Side
This is a flat, paved riverside route. It's populated with bladers, runners, cyclists, and dog-walkers, but it's free of car traffic.

Take the ramp that crosses over the FDR Drive. Start your run at 59th Street on the East Side. Head north, keeping the river on your right. The route takes you along the water's edge, and it features great views of Roosevelt Island, the Triboro Bridge, and Randall's Island. As you approach the Triboro Bridge at 120th Street, turn around at the footbridge and run back to 59th Street for a 10K (6.2-mile) run.

ACCESS:

By subway: 4, 5, 6, N, and R trains at the 59th Street and Lexington Avenue station. Walk east on 59th Street.

Running Choices from Major Tourist Neighborhoods

SOHO: Due to extremes of traffic, including delivery cyclists speeding across the roads at every conceivable angle, it is advised to take the subway up to Central Park.

HARLEM: The upper reaches of the trail that parallel the West Side Highway, and the Central Park entrance at 110th Street, are the best bets.

TRIBECA: Head for the West Side Highway.

GREENWICH VILLAGE   One of the most unusual running tracks anywhere is the wide, uninterrupted half-mile sidewalk around Washington Square Park. It's surrounded by the Village—famed for its Dylanesque ambiance and quaint restaurants. The distance is short, but the advantages of a nonstop running loop in downtown Manhattan make this a popular choice. It's entirely flat, but the only facilities are in the local coffee shops. On April First, the Backwards Mile is held around this asphalt rectangle.

Brooklyn
Prospect Park
The primary running spot in Brooklyn is Prospect Park, Brooklyn's version of Central Park. Designed by Frederick Law Olmstead and Calvert Vaux, the men who designed Manhattan's Central Park, Prospect Park is the oasis for Brooklyn's running community. There are a variety of routes, the most common being the hilly 3.35-mile road

loop. Historically, this park was the site where George Washington fought the Battle of Long Island early in the American Revolution.

Prospect Park is closed to traffic between 10 A.M. and 3 P.M., and also between 7 and 10 P.M. on weekdays during the summer. Yes, there are water fountains and public rest rooms.

ACCESS:

By subway: 2 or 5 train to Grand Army Plaza or Eastern Parkway.

D or Q train to Parkside Avenue or Prospect Park.

F train to 15th Street or Prospect Park.

Bay Ridge Bike and Pedestrian Path

This is a flat and traffic-free asphalt path through beautiful section of Southern Brooklyn, with wonderful views of the Verrazano-Narrows Bridge and New York Bay.

It can be rather windy. The total length is 2¼ miles, and there are markers every half-mile. There are water fountains and pay phones along the way.

ACCESS:

By subway: R train to 95th Street and Fort Hamilton. Walk six blocks south to John Paul Jones Park.

Sample Bay Ridge Run   Start at the foot of the Verrazano-Narrows Bridge. Follow the path with the water on your left, run to the 69th Street jetty, swing round, and double back for a 4½-mile round trip.

Dyker Beach Golf Course

The perimeter sidewalk is 2.2 miles around, mostly flat (with one big hill), and paved. There's one water fountain.

ACCESS:

McCarren Park

North Brooklyn's largest park. There's a 400m track surrounded by parkland and dirt trails; you can run loops of between ⅔ mile and 1 mile, depending on your route.

ACCESS:

Brooklyn Bridge

One of the most famous and picturesque bridges in New York, it was built late in the nineteenth century. From the Brooklyn side, there are two entrances to the Brooklyn Bridge pedestrian and bike path. The first is at the north corner of Tillary and Adams Streets in downtown Brooklyn. The concrete path starts next to the traffic entrance. From here you are about a half-mile from the beginning of the span. The second entrance is via the stairway at the corner of Prospect Street and Cadman Plaza East, just north of Cadman Plaza in Brooklyn Heights.

> "McCarren Park is mostly just a track, but I can cobble together an all-grass three-quarter-mile route along the park's fences."
>
> —Peter Krebs, Brooklyn runner

The surface is partly concrete, but in midspan it becomes a wooden boardwalk. The boardwalk is above the road, and thus the pollution from the traffic is not too bad. A painted yellow line down the middle of the boardwalk divides a bicycle lane from a walking/running lane.

On the Manhattan side, the concrete path begins across Centre Street from City Hall Park. From the Manhattan end, you can continue west across Chambers Street to Hudson River Park.

Cadman Plaza

This grassy, tree-lined park is situated at the northeast end of Brooklyn Heights, just off the Brooklyn Bridge. Run on the half-mile dirt-trail loop; it's easy on the legs, perfect for those pre-marathon easy runs. You can also run on the sidewalk that circles the park. There are water fountains at both ends.

ACCESS:

Brooklyn Heights Promenade

For splendid views of Manhattan, run to the promenade park at the western end of Brooklyn Heights.

From Cadman Plaza, head west across Cadman Plaza West, then Henry, Hicks, and Willow Streets and Columbia Heights. The Promenade is west of Columbia Heights and runs from Middagh Street at the north to Remsen Street at the south.

Red Hook Track

In Red Hook, just south of Carroll Gardens, northwest of the Park Slope neighborhood, you'll find a good Tartan running track at the City Park. (There are also football/soccer fields, baseball fields, a community swimming pool, and an indoor gym.) The track is at the corner of Columbia and Bay Streets in Red Hook, south of the Battery Tunnel entrance.

ACCESS:

> **By subway:** F or G train to 9th and Smith Streets. Go one block west to Clinton Street, south across Hamilton Avenue, then two more blocks south and west.

Staten Island

The runners of New York's largest but least-populous borough enjoy more rural runs, though they suffer from lack of variety. The key places to run in this borough are:

Clove Lakes Park

Silver Lake Park

Willowbrook Park

Great Kills Park

ACCESS:

The Staten Island Railway (SIRTOA) runs between the island's northern and southern tips, passing within a half-mile of Silver Lake and Clove Lakes parks, and right by Great Kills Park.

Clove Lakes Park

This 195-acre park is very hilly in parts, and features 3.8 miles of bridle paths and a 3.2-mile asphalt loop around the three lakes. It's traffic-free, and there's also a 2.13-mile two-lake loop.

Water fountains and bathrooms are plentiful, and in the evenings you can hear live music.

Sample Clove Lakes Park Run   Start at the double bridges near the parking lot. Run alongside the lake to the east. Cross the first bridge and turn right down the slope. Continue until you come to Martling Avenue and turn left over the bridge, following the lake. Run up the rise, and when the path flattens out you'll have a 400-meter stretch before making a left at the double bridges. Following the path round the baseball field will get you back to your starting point.

> "New York was the marathon I always wanted to win."
>
> —1992 NYC Marathon champion and Olympic silver medalist Lisa Ondieki

<u>ACCESS:</u>

By car: Cross the Verrazano-Narrows Bridge and drive down the expressway to Exit 13. Turn right at the first light onto Clove Road. Pass four lights and make a left for free parking.

By bus: From Brooklyn, take the S-53 bus to Clove Road and Victory Boulevard.

By ferry: Take the Staten Island Ferry from Battery Park in Manhattan. The park is 2½ miles from the ferry terminal. Take the S-61, S-62, S-66, or S-67 bus from the terminal to the park.

Queens

Although not the most popular borough for hotels or other accommodations, Queens offers runners a reprieve from the high Manhattan prices and is only a short commute to Midtown.

Forest Park

Most runners from this borough name Forest Park as the running hot spot. The park is almost jungle-like; it's hard to believe that you're still in New York City. There are 3.75 miles of marked hiking trails and 7 miles of bridle paths. At Victory Field is a 400-meter all-weather running track. It's also possible to run on the dirt footpath around the perimeter of the golf course. Bathrooms and water fountains are plentiful.

<u>ACCESS:</u>

By subway: J or Z train to the Woodhaven Boulevard station.

By bus: Take the Q-11 bus to Woodhaven Boulevard.

Sample Forest Park Run Start by the Woodhaven Road entrance and run east along East Main Drive for about a mile, then turn right onto Metropolitan Avenue. Turn right quickly again onto Park Lane. After about 1,000 yards, turn right on Freedom Drive. This will lead you back to East Main Drive; follow that to your starting point.

Flushing Meadow Park

Perhaps the best-known park in Queens, the 1,255-acre Flushing Meadow Park is home to Arthur Ashe Stadium and the U.S. Open tennis tournament, the Queens Museum of Art, the New York Hall of Science, Shea Stadium, the Queens Theater in the Park, and the Queens Wildlife Center. This park was also the site of the 1964 World's Fair.

A good running route is around the Meadow Lake on the tarmac path. Bathrooms, water fountains, food, telephones, and bicycle rentals are available.

ACCESS:

By subway: 7 train to Willets Point/Shea Stadium

By car: Take the Grand Central Parkway to the Flushing Meadows Corona Park exit.

Alley Pond Park

571 acres of woods, parkland, and beautiful trails. Amenities include bathrooms, water fountains, and telephones.

ACCESS:

By car: Exit the Grand Central Parkway at the Winchester/Alley Pond exit and use the parking lot.

The Bronx
Van Cortlandt Park
1,100 acres of rolling parkland in the north of the city, a half-hour subway ride from the center of Manhattan. The famously hilly cross-country course is too tough for pre-marathon runs, but there's also a 1½-mile packed-gravel running path around the periphery of the playing-field area. It's all traffic-free. For the non-running companion, there is a superb golf course, soccer fields, horse stables, and many other outdoor sporting activities.

ACCESS:

By subway: 1 train to the last stop, 242nd Street. Then walk north (the direction that the train was traveling) for ten blocks.

By car: Parking spaces are plentiful along Broadway, which borders the park. The Henry Hudson Parkway cuts through the park making directions from the city simple.

By bus: Take Bx-3, Bx-7, or Bx-9.

Sample Van Cortlandt Park Run   To begin the 5-kilometer loop, start at the seating area opposite 252nd Street. Run south on the gravel path, swing left around the large white pole at the end of the field, and head for the next white pole, approximately 200 meters ahead. Take a left around this pole, and follow the edge of the grass field until you see a gravel path to your right. It is here that the hilly trails begin. (To keep on the flat, continue straight ahead and loop the large playing-field area.) Follow the dirt path as it winds its way up and down the hills. After ¾ of a mile, take a right at the bridge, then an immediate right when exiting the bridge. Follow this path as it loops around for one mile before bringing you back to the same bridge. After recrossing the bridge, turn right, and run down the hill and back onto the playing fields. Keep right on the gravel path to finish the loop.

Riverdale Park

This small park, with asphalt trails, runs by the Hudson, not far from Van Cortlandt Park.

ACCESS:

By subway: 1 train, to 232nd Street and head west.

By bus   Take Bx-9 to 242nd Street.

The New York Botanical Gardens

A stunningly peaceful contrast to the grind of the city, these gardens are a must to visit and a delight to run in. The road loop, 2½ miles around, is closed to public traffic and a feeder to the many trails that run through the park. The terrain is undulating and the air is good except for those who suffer from hay fever!

The Gardens are open from Tuesday to Sunday, 10 A.M. to 6 P.M., although between November and March the park closes at 4 P.M.

Long Island

Bethpage Bike Path

The recommended spot to run in Long Island, this is a marked asphalt path that goes on for miles, with options to run off-road through plentiful parkland. It's well marked every 400 meters, and runs from Merrick Road in Massapequa to the Bethpage State Park picnic grounds. From south to north, it passes through the Massapequa Park Preserve, parallels the Bethpage Parkway, then skirts the golf course and enters the park grounds. It is predominantly flat except in the state park, where there are a few rolling hills. Water fountains and restrooms are available at the train station and at the golf clubhouse, approximately five miles from the starting point.

For group runs on the bike path every Saturday and Sunday morning, call the Massapequa Road Runners Club, Alex Flyntz, (516) 796–1900.

ACCESS:

By train: Long Island Rail Road (LIRR) to Massapequa Station.

Westchester County

A mere thirty-minute train ride will take you to a rural running retreat—the Rockefeller Estate. It is here that the current men's world record-holder for the marathon, Khalid Khannouchi, lives and trains. There are miles and miles of beautiful running trails in Rockefeller State Park. However, it is very easy to get lost, as the trails are numerous and extend for many miles.

Chapter Six

Food in the City

Most runners love to eat, and if you're one who does, you'll probably love New York. It's been said that you can eat three meals a day in New York restaurants, without ever visiting the same place, forever! (By the time you'd gotten through all the eateries, plenty of new ones would have opened.) For your much briefer stay during Marathon Week, you'll still have time for some great dining experiences—but make sure that they help your race, not hinder it.

New York Dining Tips

■ Check the prices; two restaurants may share the same building but be a world apart in price. New York is America's most expensive city in which to dine, and some NYC eateries have the kind of prices that you'd expect on a luxury yacht. However, bargains can be found, especially if you cut out the wine!

■ Check first to see how smoke-free (if that's your preference) the smoke-free zone actually is. Space costs big money in New York, and proximity to a "portioned off" area often means falling victim to foul air.

■ New Yorkers typically eat later than people in most other cities; expect the "rush" to be somewhat later than elsewhere.

■ Call first about any special needs you may have (wheelchair access, baby-stroller access, etc.).

■ If you make a reservation, be punctual. Nothing riles the staff more than a party who turn up a half-hour late expecting their table to still be held. The clock never stops in New York! But even so . . .

■ If the place is popular, expect a wait. In NYC, there's a good chance that the meal will be worth it.

■ The average tip for a competent waitperson is 18 percent; in NYC anything below 15 percent will be met with disdain. Although you can make your own choice, remember that tips do "pay" the wait staff. If you have a complaint, make yourself heard.

Restaurant Guides touts New York as a premier dining city. The week before the race might not be the best time to overindulge every night, but you should still be able to enjoy and appreciate this aspect of NYC without jeopardizing your performance.

Virtually every neighborhood in the city has wonderful restaurants; here's a small selection that has been chosen for runner-friendly reasons (not-too-long seating waits; generally smoke-free air; and healthy, generous portions):

Bagels

NYC is the home of the bagel, the breakfast choice of runners nation-wide. It's a New York tradition to follow a long training run with a bagel and coffee. Hence a comprehensive list of some of the best bagel eateries in the city is necessary. If you do nothing else in New York, make sure that you follow at least one training run with a bagel and coffee—then you will have truly experienced the New York Run!

Au Bon Pain
Fifth Avenue and 14th Street
Bagels in a fast-food–style café setting. For the non-bagel eater, there are many other alternatives, though if you're not here for the bagels, then . . . The lunchtime rush makes this downtown meeting spot a crowded and bumpy one. The house specialty, for those craving a sweet-tooth fix, must be the Dutch-apple bagel.

Bagels on the Square
7 Carmine Street, near Sixth Avenue
"Salt bagels." This strange variation is the house specialty in this West Village bagelry with a friendly staff. Garlic and onion models are also top-notch. Huge bagels, and they're nice and fresh.

Ess-A-Bagel
First Avenue and 21st Street
Thick, dense, doughy bagels. Questionable coffee. Typical table-talk centers around complaints about the service. Recommended is the lox multi-grain.

Ess-A-Bagel
Third Avenue between 50th and 51st Streets

Bigger, fatter bagels than at most other places in Midtown. To avoid the invariably long lines, go directly to the back counter for bagels only. Can be extremely crowded at lunch hour. The poppyseed bagel wins best-of-the-bunch at this establishment.

Gramercy Bagels
Third Avenue between 20th and 21st Streets

Basically a bagel café, and never too crowded—a huge plus for this part of town. The bagels are a little crustier than at the usual bagelry. The size is good, and the taste is up there, too.

Only cinnamon-raisin and sesame have been sampled to date, the former scoring highly, the latter a little *too* crusty.

Healthy Bagel
Second Avenue between 71st and 72nd Streets

Sourdough bagels are the specialty. Baked only on weekends are unique cranberry-raisin-walnut sourdough bagels—quite a treat. Bagel enthusiasts often make long treks for the always-available sourdough-raisin bagels. Other unusual flavors: rye, herb, and challah.

The walls of this eatery are literally covered with celebrity pictures, and it offers a typical deli menu at moderate prices.

Hot Bagels
Brooklyn Heights on Montague Street

The poppyseed bagels from this eatery in Brooklyn are recommended by many. According to Anke Dieker from Munnich, Germany, this is *the* place to stop after running over the Brooklyn Bridge.

Hot and Crusty Bagels
Lexington Avenue between 85th and 86th Streets

Good-sized, fancy, and flavorful authentic bagels.

Lenny's Bagels
Broadway and 98th Street

Great variety of interesting bagels—the Bad Boy and the Uptown, to name a couple.* The staff come from the four corners of the globe, and the change you're given is often more or less than the amount you should receive.

Murray's Bagels
Sixth Avenue and 13th Street

A tip from local runner Michelle Rossettie, a 2:50 marathoner: "Whenever I go into Murray's, I ask which varieties are warm or about to come out of the oven, and that's what I get." And the flavor to hope for? "A multigrain bagel—with peanut butter and jelly."

Pick-A-Bagel
Second Avenue and 77th Street

In the bread-for-the-buck department, this place wins dough-down. Huge bagels of a chewy consistency make it a runner's retreat. [Frequented by the W&W,] it's packed on Sunday mornings. The staff are efficient and speedy, but the atmosphere is rather sterile, so pick up the bagels and eat them at your hotel.

Russ and Daughters
179 East Houston Street, between First Avenue, Allen Street, and Orchard Street

Says Australian runner Jenny Hailstone, "I'm not a huge fan of bagels (they're too doughy for my taste) but the bialys from Lower East Side landmark Russ and Daughters are worth buying in bulk." A crispier, lighter, less filling cousin of the bagel, bialys are flatter, and instead of a hole, they have an indentation full of onion paste in the middle.

Author's Choice Try the New Horizon, with flaxseeds and raisins, or the Ali Baba with chocolate and raisins. Buy a dozen and get six free!

Tal Bagels

333 East 86th Street between First and Second Avenues

Good bagels, a wide variety of interesting spreads, lightning-fast service, and lots of seating. The coffee at this bagelry gets a good rating, too!

The Bagelry

3rd Avenue and 30th Street

Smaller and crustier bagels than most, and a denser texture. Try the flat bagel—"squashed before baking." Apparently, malt is used in place of sugar to impart a distinct flavor.

Recommended? A toasted pumpernickel or whole-wheat bagel with sundried tomato cream cheese and a slice of onion.

The Bagelry

96th Street and Madison Avenue

Not to be confused with the previous listing. The bagels are small, smaller and *the* smallest in New York. With a hickory taste to the coffee and less-than-fresh bagels on the counter, this bagelry went on the not-to-be-visited-again list!

Recommended? Picking another place.

The Green Tree

Madison Avenue and 89th Street

The key attraction to this deli is its closeness to the NYRR headquarters and Central Park. The bagels taste "imported"—definitely not baked freshly on the premises. Steer clear of the plain bagel, as it is rather dry. To be recommended: the cinnamon-raisin and the sesame. Cream cheese is plastered on by the pint; be sure to ask for a shovel to reduce the bounteous slab. The deli's prices are reasonable.

Coffee

In a word: Starbucks. New York has a tradition of strong coffee, and perhaps that's why Starbucks has proved conspicuously popular in the city. On almost every block, the green sign is there—with the delicious aroma of the coffee bean floating nearby. However, there is a catch! The bagels are yet to match the coffee. A solution is to buy bagels elsewhere, then plant yourself at Starbucks. For this tester, the staff have never complained about the imported food! The coffee prices at Starbucks are a little higher than at a local deli, but the taste is consistently excellent, making it well worth the extra cents. The locations are too numerous to list; check out the Starbucks website at www.starbucks.com.

Pizza

Although the Italians may differ, many cite New York as the pizza capital of the world. This is great news for runners, as a pizza provides excellent fuel. If you stay away from the extra cheeses and the pepperoni and eat a pizza with vegetable toppings, you have a near-perfect meal. Below are a few of New York's finest pizza parlors.

Arturo's
106 West Houston Street; (212) 475-9828
Long waits and a tiny location make this pizzeria unpopular for the marathoner at peak hours. But the crowds are there for a reason: great pizza! The rest of the menu is somewhat lacking, but the pizza is truly majestic—possibly even magisterial. Go for the plain cheese-and-tomato variety, the New Yorker's choice. There's a bar to make the waits a little more pleasant.

Denino's Pizzeria/Tavern

524 Port Richmond Avenue, Staten Island; (718) 442-9401

This family-style, sit-down pizza parlor is short on atmosphere, but its legendary thin-crust pies are first-class. The "Garbage Pie," an assortment of sausage, mushrooms, meatballs, onion, and pepperoni, is definitely not the recipe for marathon success; stick to the plain—it's a classic.

Grimaldi's

19 Old Fulton Street, Brooklyn; (718) 858-4300

One of NYC's most famous pizzerias, it's always winning awards. But expect long waits—even when the restaurant doesn't appear full! Some say it's the Brooklyn way.

John's Pizza

Four locations: 278 Bleecker Street, 260 West 44th Street, 408 East 64th Street, and 48 West 65th Street, (212) 243-1680

Always ranked highly in any city's guide for pizza. Thin crust can, for some, be a little too thin—sometimes a burnt bit on the side. The ambiance is that of a fast-food diner. Late hours help with the rating; beware that the Bleecker Street venue does not accept credit cards.

Joe's Pizza

7 Carmine Street & 233 Bleecker Street; (212) 366-1182

Cheap but excellent food, located in the Village district. A line up pay, and eat pizzeria with no frills.

"The best in New York—no question!" swears marathon runner and true New Yorker Ben "Pizza" Kessler. Late hours; no credit cards accepted.

La Pizza Fresca Ristorante

31 East 20th Street; (212) 598-0141

Certified by the Italian government as "vera pizza Napoletana" (true Neapolitan pizza)—one of only two restaurants in NYC to win this award. An upscale pizzeria with great flavors; the pasta dishes are also very good.

Totonno's

1524 Neptune Avenue, Brooklyn; (718) 372-8606

Established in 1924 by Anthony "Totonno" Pero, this Coney Island pizzeria is the country's oldest pizza joint that's been run continuously by the same family. Try the signature white pizza made with mozzarella, pecorino Romano, and fresh garlic for a truly unique NYC dining experience. Delivery isn't available. The Manhattan Totonno's, at 1544 Second Avenue, (212) 327-2800, features a full pasta menu in addition to the pizza.

Two Boots

Four locations: 37 Avenue A, 74 Bleecker Street, 201 West 11th Street, and 514 2nd Street in Brooklyn; (212) 505-2276

Great prices and Cajun-style pizzas. (The "two boots" are Italy and Louisiana.) A student hangout with adventurous but really tasty flavors. There's a large assortment of other good foods.

V & T Pizzeria

1024 Amsterdam Avenue; (212) 663-1708

Cheap and cheesy, and in generous sizes. Also available are enormous portions of stuffed shells, baked ziti, veal parmigiana, baked clams, and classic spaghetti with meatballs. A popular choice for university students, with late-night serving hours.

HOW TO SPEAK AND EAT LIKE A NEW YORKER

"Ax"	ask
Bialy	like an underbaked holeless bagel
Knish	Jewish potato roll with onion, sold traditionally at football games. (Say "Ka-nish.")
"Jeet?"	Did you eat?
Schmear	small amount of cream cheese spread on a bagel
Yo!	A term used to attract the waitperson

Hamburgers

Americans eat three burgers per week on average. New Yorkers probably hike up that quota. Some recommended burger restaurants:

Cafeteria
119 Seventh Avenue; (212) 414-1717
24-hour Chelsea burger heaven.

Corner Bistro
331 West 4th Street; (212) 242-9502
Legendary for its inexpensive NYC burgers. A must-visit establishment in the West Village.

Island Burgers & Shakes
766 Ninth Avenue; (212) 307-7934
Right in the heart of Manhattan. Cheap but highly rated. Credit
cards not accepted.

Jackson Hole
Multiple locations; (212) 679-3264
Marathon-sized portions and reasonable prices, always ranked high
among NYC burger restaurants. The fast staff turnover can sometimes
result in sloppy service.

Joe Allen
326 West 46th Street; (212) 581-6464
In the theater district, with reasonable prices and late hours.

Diner

85 Broadway, Brooklyn; (718) 486-3077

American with French flavor to please all palates.

Union Square Café

21 East 16th Street; (212) 243-4020

Very popular and with higher-than-usual prices, but the burgers here are sublime.

Italian

There are literally hundreds of good Italian restaurants in New York City, and that's good news for the runner. Pastas and tomato-based sauces are just the recipe for running success. Five runner-friendly restaurants are:

Baci Italian

7107 Third Avenue, Brooklyn; (718) 836-5536

Beautiful, quaint borough restaurant with great food and big portions at moderate prices.

Café Fiorello

1900 Broadway; (212) 595-5330

Great pastas. Rather crowded before theater curtains. Very good thin-crust pizza, too.

Da Silvano

260 Sixth Avenue; (212) 982-2342

Not cheap, but very good food, including great bread.

Pomodoro Rosso

229 Columbus Avenue; (212) 721-3009

Some of the best Italian food in NYC. Great table bread and gigantic portions ensure that no one leaves this restaurant feeling hungry.

Teodora
141 East 57th Street; (212) 826-7101
Friendly; not too expensive; and fresh, tasty ingredients.

American

America
9 East 18th Street; (212) 505-2110
Run-of-the-mill American-style eatery, a fast turnover with moderate prices.

Hard Rock Café
221 West 57th Street; (212) 489-6565
Good-quality fast food, and lots to look at while-u-wait.

Junior's
386 Flatbush Avenue, Brooklyn; (718) 852-5257
Cheap, huge portions, and the best cheesecake ever. World-famous, or nearly! Worth the journey over the bridge.

Park Avalon
225 Park Avenue South; (212) 533-2500
Good music, food, and decor make this classy restaurant a winner.

The Water Club
500 East 30th Street; (212) 683-3333
Great views over the East River from this barge restaurant; good American food, but at a price. Lots of nice table bread for the hungry runner.

More Great Restaurants in the Outer Boroughs

Staten Island

Trattoria Romana

1476 Hylan Boulevard; (718) 980-3113

Great hearty Italian meals, perfect for the pre-race carbo-eating.

Aesop's Tables

1233 Bay Street (718) 720-2005

Nice quaint restaurant with reasonable prices and good food. The service is top notch, and there is also a great garden for the "summer weather" days. Definitely one of the better finds on Staten Island.

The Bronx

Roberto's

632 East 186th Street; (718) 733-9503

Great Italian uptown food, generous portions, and the bread never stops coming. A great pasta-loading restaurant.

Lobster Box

34 City Island Avenue; (718) 885-1952

Many make pilgrimages to this specialty lobster restaurant known for its great seafood and nice setting. Worth a drive.

Queens

Uncle George's

33-19 Broadway; (718) 626-0593

A Greek restaurant with low prices and fresh food.

Cooking with Jazz

12-01 154th Street; (718) 767-6979

As the name suggests, a Cajun flavor. Good food, and moderate prices to boot!

Brooklyn

Marco Polo

345 Court Street; (718) 852-5015

Great reliable Italian diner. Superb ratings for the hungry athlete, with tasty pasta dishes galore at reasonable prices.

Rasputin

2670 Coney Island Avenue; (718) 332-8111

Authentic Russian restaurant, and a show with the meal. Perhaps not the place to go before the race, but for post-race lavish dining, it should be an option.

Finding Ethnic Cuisines in NYC

There are many ethnic enclaves in New York where a particular cuisine is common. Here are some of them; to find authentic food, a good method is to step inside the establishment and look around. If there are people in the seating area who you can tell are from the country that the restaurant purports to represent, you can bet the food is the real thing.

Indian	Head for East 6th Street, called Little India for its many excellent restaurants.
Chinese	Obviously, Chinatown in Lower Manhattan.
Italian	Little Italy in lower Manhattan, although typically there are great Italian restaurants throughout the city.
French	Upper West Side, Midtown.

South American/ Mexican	Upper, *upper* East Side (Spanish Harlem) starting at 110th Street
Brazilian	Midtown Manhattan

Chapter Seven

Getting to the Start

The best method of getting to the starting line of the NYC Marathon is to take one of the official race buses that leave from both the New York City Public Library at Fifth Avenue and 42nd Street and the Continental Airlines Arena at the Meadowlands Sports Complex in New Jersey. Purchase a bus ticket by checking the box on the official entry form—this service costs $6 and is money well spent. This is your special day; don't mess up at the last hurdle. Leave early on race day to make one of these destinations with time to spare. The buses begin transporting runners at 5:30 A.M. from the Fifth Avenue location and 6 A.M. from the Meadowlands. They stop running after 7:30 A.M., period! For runners needing wheelchair assistance, wheelchair-accessible buses will leave from the Fifth Avenue location (between 36th and 39th Streets). It's advisable to ask at the number pick-up for an exact location for athletes with disabilities.

Runners can make the journey to the start by car, but be warned: The Verazzano Bridge closes to traffic at 9 A.M., and parking is extremely difficult to find near the starting line. However, as a last resort if you miss the buses, take a taxi and ask for the marathon start in

> "The worst feeling before the marathon is when you are stressed from being late for the event. I like to arrive early—at least two hours before the event—so I can sit down and relax and concentrate on the marathon."
>
> —1990 champion Douglas Wakiihuri

Staten Island. (For $30 you can take car service.) Many runners prefer to take the bus service, as new friendships are made and the excitement truly begins as you sit amongst your fellow competitors.

Race Day

On the morning of the race day, make sure you have at least two alarms set to wake you. You mustn't oversleep on this day! Double-check with your hotel desk if requesting a wake-up call, and ask a friend to give you a call, too, just in case.

Aim to wake up earlier than necessary, and have your running clothes and baggage laid out and pre-checked the night before the marathon. People often forget important items in the early-morning hours! Again, talking to a friend who is also running can help here; compare your must-take items.

Eat a breakfast of 400 to 600 calories about four hours before the race. Here's one suggested breakfast:

A banana

Four pieces of white toast with jelly

A cup of coffee or tea

A bottle of sports drink

When asked what scientifically balanced foods he ate before his centennial Boston Marathon victory, Moses Tanui replied, "I just had toast and tea." Plain and simple gets the job done.

Use the bathroom before departing. This task will usually have to be repeated a few times; don't worry—this is completely normal. In fact, don't be shocked at the starting line if you see many runners continuing to "squat"—or discreetly use bottles—right up to the very last possible moment before the starting cannon fires. (If you can't manage that, don't be alarmed—there are Porta Potties along the whole course.)

PROFILE
Allan Steinfeld, Race Director

One could say that Allan Steinfeld was born for the job of New York City Marathon Race Director: He entered the world on Fifth Avenue, in a hospital that's actually on the course! Allan has been involved with the NYRR and the marathon since their inceptions. A former 22-second 200-meter runner, he is no slouch on his feet, and yes, he has run a marathon, albeit not New York's—he has certain obligations that day!

Steinfeld's marathon expertise is not limited to New York: He was the chief referee for the men's and women's Olympic Marathons in Los Angeles in 1984. He is also the president of Running USA and vice president of the global Association of International Marathons, and he holds a Masters degree from Cornell University.

He can often be found running on the reservoir in Central Park.

How to Dress for the Marathon

You'll notice that the top runners at nearly all marathons are dressed in singlets and shorts. However, these runners have been allowed an adequate warmup, are usually allowed to keep their warmup suits on until minutes before the starting horn, and don't have to stand still for very long at the starting line.

Many factors should help determine your dress code for the marathon, and some changes may be made even after you've started the race.

When it's cold, the body takes a long time to warm up properly. The golden rule for pre-race attire is that it's a lot easier to discard extra clothes than to run cold wishing you had dressed a little more conservatively. The starting line and the first couple of miles of the course are always littered with discarded items of clothing. Dress to discard!

The basics are the classic singlet and shorts. Likely additions are a T-shirt, either long- or short-sleeved and preferably made from a microfiber material (such as CoolMax), a windbreaker, gloves, and a hat. Take all these clothes with you to the starting line to keep your options open.

If the temperature is between 25° and 45° F: Consider wearing a long-sleeved T-shirt under your singlet. Also consider wearing a thin pair of tights, made specifically for runners (so they won't chafe). You'll probably want to start out with gloves and a hat.

For between 45° and 55° F: Wear a singlet or T-shirt. Consider starting in a sweatshirt that you can discard after a few miles. Shorts, or short tights, should be sufficient. Gloves and a hat aren't essential, but you might wear a pair of thin gloves to discard along the way.

For 60° F and above: singlet and shorts, and a short-sleeved T-shirt to discard just before the gun sounds.

> "The starting line of the New York City Marathon is kind of a giant time bomb behind you about to go off. It is the most spectacular start in sport."
>
> —Bill Rodgers,
> three-time NYC Marathon winner

Special considerations are rain, heat, and bright sunshine.

For rain, you might want a light waterproof windbreaker, and maybe a cap to keep the water out of your eyes.

For the sun, consider sunglasses, and be sure to apply sunscreen to your face and shoulders.

For high heat, wear light-colored clothing, which will repel the heat rather than absorb it. A lightweight white hat with a brim is a good idea.

All clothes discarded at the starting line are donated to charity!

The Starting Area

There are actually three starting lines: Blue, Red, and Green.

The Blue group runs along the right half of the Verrazano's upper level. The elite men start at the front of this group.

The Red group runs along the left half of the upper level. The women runners are in this group, with the invited women at the head. This group appears to have a head start on the other two areas, but the course evens out in Brooklyn.

The Green group runs along the left half of the bridge's lower level. The local elite men are at the head of this group.

The right side of the bridge's lower level is used for traffic. The three groups are kept separate for a few miles. (Don't cross any barriers to try to join another group!) By Mile 8, the three groups have merged.

The organizers don't appreciate the problems that occur when runners switch numbers or try to get to a different-colored starting area. You've been given your start for a reason, and the field's groups are balanced in number. If you really want to run with someone who will be in a different starting corral, you can arrange to meet at the 8-mile marker at a certain time if one of you will be on the Red start, or earlier at the 4-mile marker if the two of you have a Green and Blue color combination.

The ChampionChip

With your race number you will be loaned a small, circular, plastic timing chip.

This device helps the organizers of the event tremendously. Be sure to follow the package instructions on how to affix the chip to your shoe.

With "the Chip," results are available instantaneously. Furthermore, the Chips can be read at checkpoints along the course, updating officials as to the runners' progress.

When the runner crosses the starting line, the device is activated, and at the finishing line it is read and deactivated, recording a net time. If you are unfortunate and have to start at the very back of the field, it could be quite a few minutes before you even reach the starting line. Thus your "gun" starting time will be that much slower. But the Chip will record the exact amount of time that it takes you to travel between the starting line and the finish line. However, to win the race you'll still have to be the first across the finish line, as the gun times are used for overall placement. (Otherwise, it would be impossible to tell which runner was in the lead, and a cunning competitor could wait ten seconds after the gun before crossing the mat and, theoretically, win by finishing nine seconds behind the first runner to cross the line.)

More good news is that your net time will count toward qualifying for an automatic entry to both the following year's New York City and Boston marathons.

The Chip has also helped officials catch cheats whose recordings are mysteriously missing at a checkpoint. A race organizer will often place a Chip mat at an unexpected point on the course to check that all runners complete the distance. Backed up with video cameras, the Chip greatly reduces the cheater's odds of "winning."

Each Chip has a transponder that's linked to an individual number and runner. When the runner crosses a rubberized mat that can record and transmit encrypted data, a signal is sent to a computer base.

The advantage of the Chip is that it eliminates the need for chute finishes, where the runners have to line up in their finishing order. Results are available as the runners cross the finish line, and can include intermediate times from various points on the course.

There are a couple of disadvantages. If your Chip falls off your shoe, not only will your finish go unrecorded, but you must pay for the loss (currently $30). Also, if there is a system breakdown, there is no manual backup plan.

Therefore, make sure that your Chip is securely fastened to your running shoe, and when you finish, make sure that a race volunteer clips your Chip.

Make sure your chip will not cause you any discomfort while running. One runner incorrectly tied the Chip to the tongue of her shoe, causing a blister to form. Follow the instructional diagram provided with the Chip.

If you like, you can buy your own personal ChampionChip at New York Road Runners. Then you'll have your own number to use at most international running events time and time again.

How to Survive at the Start

At the staging area before the marathon start, the first thing most runners do is line up for the Porta Potties. It's a good idea to bring your own toilet paper, as supplies always seem short.

Next, it could be time to grab some coffee, or at least some water. Some people wait this long before eating breakfast, and if you're hungry it's not a bad idea to join them. Bagels and yogurt are popular choices.

Milk, yogurt, coffee, Gatorade, fruit juice, and spring water are available at the athletes' village at Fort Wadsworth from 6 to 10 A.M.

Be careful with the coffee; too much can keep you running back to the Porta Potties. This is one morning when you don't want to swallow too many diuretics.

Try to find an area to sit below one of the weatherproof tents—even if it's not raining. (It's better to be prepared.) Take a plastic bag to sit on, to keep your clothes dry if the ground is damp. (It usually is!)

Between 8:30 A.M. and 9 A.M., religious services are held at the Fort Wadsworth athletes' village.

It's advisable to walk to your corral at 10 A.M. or soon afterward. First, place anything that you want to retrieve at the finishing line in the provided UPS bag. Look for the table—they're alphabetized by last name—where volunteers will load your bag onto one of the many buses that transport them to Manhattan. It may seem impossible that you'll ever see your bag again, but the chances are excellent that you will—very, very few bags get lost. However, it's not wise to leave any valuables in these bags.

The streams of runners walking to the corrals make navigation easy. Your registration card will have told you whether you'll be on the Red, Green, or Blue start. Signage should show you clearly where to walk. Upon reaching the corrals, most runners are nervous and chat incessantly. Stick to your game plan; don't suddenly decide to switch tactics and run with a stranger just because his advice seems interesting. Discard any last-minute clothes, and apply Vaseline to the areas that might rub: under the arms, in the groin, and for women, along the seams of your jogging bra.

At 10:45 A.M., the national anthem is sung.

The elite women start at 10:50; you have 25 minutes to let the fast ladies get a head start!

At 11:15 the main race begins! Wait for the starting cannon—the time seems to fly by! When the cannon sounds, try to move slowly and carefully. Don't get frustrated if you can't get into your stride for the first few minutes. Patience is a virtue in the marathon, and frustration is only wasted energy.

The 2002 NYCM followed the lead of the London Marathon by instituting separate starting times for the elite men and women racers. The feedback from the elite women was totally positive. Marathon debutant and Olympian Marla Runyan, "I'm very pleased that New York has adopted this policy." Joyce Chepchumba, who set a marathon world best in a women's only field underlined the obvious: "A women's record should only be allowed without male assistance, like in a track race." Obviously, the TV viewing is enhanced, as viewers get a much clearer picture of the unfolding women's race. No longer can a female runner slip away unnoticed from her competitors, "hidden" in a huddle of male runners. Women starting in the main field are not eligible for the overall prize; the female winner is the first from the elite starting group. Moreover, the chances of an unknown female running a 2:20 marathon are infinitesimal in this day and age. All sub-2:40 females should contact the race director if they wish to be considered for the elite field. This should be done in writing well before the event.

Early Starts

For athletes with disabilities who need extra time, an early start is available at 8:50 A.M. at the Blue start. The wheelchair/hand-crank start for the official qualifying division is held at 10:20 A.M. at the Green start.

Last-Minute Reminders

- Don't try any fad diets in the last few days before the race. Protein, carbohydrates, and fat are equally necessary for a balanced energy metabolism during a marathon race. Just try to shift the emphasis toward carbohydrates for the last few days.

■ Don't eat any solids in the last two hours before the race, unless you're used to the feeling of running with food in your stomach.

■ Eat a light breakfast, preferably of cereals, toast, or a bagel, with tea or coffee—whatever is familiar. Stay away from fatty foods and hard-to-digest proteins.

■ Refrain from using antiperspirants or beauty products. They'll clog up your pores and stop your skin from "breathing" while you run.

■ Wear only your tried-and-tested shoes and clothes for the race. Don't wear that new shirt that you bought at the Expo the day before!

■ Dress in a running outfit that's suitable for the conditions of the day.

■ Make sure there are no foreign objects in your shoes.

■ Double-knot your shoelaces, and jog a few steps to ensure that there is no movement.

■ Don't forget the Vaseline.

■ Try not to run around too much before the start. By the time you're in the corral, any previous jogging warmup will be negated, as standing still in a packed crowd of thousands of runners will drop your heart rate back to normal, and your legs will tighten up from the jogging. It's a better idea to treat the opening mile or two of the race as a warmup. However, if it's possible, try to stretch a little in the last twenty minutes.

Chapter Eight

Spectating: Where to Watch the Runners

There are a number of different ways to view the marathon, depending on your energy levels and your needs.

The most relaxed method may be to sit in front of the television in a pair of sneakers and hope the race runs past your hotel window. This could happen, if you were to stay at the Essex House on Central Park South, for instance.

One step further is to pick a location on the course, travel there, and watch the whole race go by. Recommended spots would be Mile 8 for Brooklynites, Miles 16 and 22 through 26 for Manhattanites, Mile 20 for Bronx spectators, and Mile 14 in Queens. The advantages of this method over the hotel-slouch technique are many. The energy of the runners can really be felt from the ground level.

The third idea is to travel via subway to a number of different locations at which to watch the race. This is by far the most exciting way to see the marathon, though it is also the most tiring. The main disadvantage of this plan is that it only really works if you are watching the race as a whole, or looking out for one friend, or two of similar speed. You won't be able to wait around to cheer for the whole team; pretty much as soon as your runner passes by it will be time to get back to the sub-way station to reach the next viewing point.

A compromise is to pick two viewing spots. Below, we'll look at some different plans.

The Hotel Slouch's Guide

Most imperative for the spectating slouch is to get an accommodation on the route itself—if possible, with a window that opens out onto the course. This qualifies you as "being there."

Buy some Gatorade, if you'd like the flavor of being on the course. Tune in to WNBC for full race coverage from 10 A.M. through 3 P.M. When the runners approach, stick your head out the window (if it opens) and yell your support.

Anyone more interested in interacting with the race than the confirmed hotel slouch (and we've seldom seen a truly fulfilled hotel slouch) can use this list:

SPECTATOR ESSENTIALS

- Umbrella and/or rain clothes

- Camera

- Money

- Watch (stopwatch-equipped is a plus)

- Food and drinks, for you and any running friend

- This guide book!

The One-Spot Guide

The main drawback to this plan is that if you're trying to spot one runner you could easily miss him or her. But if you pick a premium spot, the advantages are many: There's no pressure to get anywhere at a certain time, you can enjoy seeing the fastest to the slowest pass by, and you'll enjoy being part of the supporting crowd around you. A drawback could be the weather; dress warmly and take rain clothing.

The Two-Spot Guide

New York's winding course makes it possible—and popular—to watch the race from two points. (In Boston, for comparison, where the marathon runs from point to point on a nearly straight line, this is far more difficult.)

By far the easiest plan for those in Manhattan is to watch the race go by on First Avenue from somewhere between 72nd and 86th Streets, and then walk west to Central Park and watch the runners go by again between the 23- and 24-mile marks. An advantage here is that you don't have to rely on public transport to get you to your second spot. The walk is about three-quarters of a mile, and the marathoners must run seven miles. Even if your runner is a super-fast Kenyan at the front of the pack, you'll have more than half an hour to make the short trip from First Avenue to Central Park. You should make it with time to spare.

A more adventurous step is to choose a viewing point early on, say in Brooklyn, and then take the subway in to Manhattan to catch the race at a later point. The main advantage of this idea over all other plans is that you could conceivably go to, say, Mile 4 and watch the entire field, from the first runner to the last, and then head to Central Park South to watch them all again.

The Multi-Spot Plan

For the active supporter, it is very possible to view the marathon at a number of points with the cunning use of the New York subway system.

Be warned—you will have an active day. But the benefits are a tour of the boroughs, seeing the runners through the gradual stages of the race's progress, and a chance to see your runner or runners again if you miss them at one stage.

Here's a tried-and-true plan for an optimum *five* viewing points.

■ Begin by taking the R train to the 86th Street Station in Brooklyn. This is a tough spot visually, as the runners arrive in droves. Don't be disappointed if you miss seeing a particular runner at this early stage. You'll definitely get the full impression of the massive field at one of the earliest possible viewing spots.

■ Hop back down the subway and ride the R back to Pacific Street, still in Brooklyn. You're now near the 8-mile mark. (Use the tips listed earlier to make sure your runner can also spot you.) Remember, the marathon is said to be 60 percent training and 40 percent mental—it's imperative that you, the supporter, greet your runner with the most positive attitude you can muster!

■ After you've seen who you want to see, this is a good time to pop into one of the nearby delis to grab lunch before the next stop.

■ There is a walk-thru from the Pacific Street station to the Atlantic Avenue station. Follow the directions for the Manhattan-bound 4 and 5 trains; the numbers will be circled in green. Take this subway to the 59th Street and Lexington Avenue station in Manhattan.

■ Walk the three blocks east to First Avenue, where the runners will experience one of the highlights of the marathon—the huge, loud crowd welcoming the runners to Manhattan at the 16-mile mark. Virtually every runner feels great at this point—people have likened the experience to running into a capacity-crowd stadium as a member of the home team. Due to the densely packed spectators, you may have problems making contact with your runner(s). Never mind; at the next destination it will be much easier.

■ Walk back to the Lexington Avenue station and take the 4 train uptown to the 138th Street station. You are now just past the 20-mile mark. The crowds are sparse, but it is here that your runner will need you the most. You will be able to be seen easily and to hand anything to your runners that they might need, such as a bottle of sport drink, a dry T-shirt, or an energy-gel packet. This is also a good photo opportunity, because the runners are spread out—and many are moving a bit more slowly!

■ Walk back to the 138th Street station, and take the 4 train back to the 59th Street station, then transfer to the N or R train heading toward Brooklyn, *not* toward Queens. Get out at the second stop, 57th Street and Seventh Avenue. Walk two blocks north to Central Park South, one of the most prestigious addresses in New York. You are at the 25½-mile point! This section of the course will most likely be chockablock with

> In 1980, Ernest Condor ran the entire New York City Marathon backwards!

spectators when you arrive; walking east toward Fifth Avenue may allow for better viewing. Alternatively, you can walk west toward Columbus Circle. The marathoners have only a kilometer to go from Central Park South, and they radiate a great aura of accomplishment—and exhaustion. They are about three minutes from becoming New York City Marathon finishers!

■ From Columbus Circle, at Central Park South and Eighth Avenue, you can walk north on Central Park West (the continuation of Eighth Avenue north of 59th Street) about three-quarters of a mile to the Family Reunion Area and see your running friends one more time!

After this marathon subway journey, you can say that you've experienced the marathon as thoroughly as possible without running it yourself—and the day will have flown by.

All outdoor spectators are advised to wear warm and comfortable clothes, with a waterproof windbreaker available as the outer layer. If you're hoping to be spotted by a competing friend, wear a distinctive block color, the brighter the better.

Make a game plan and decide where you'll be at what time. If you're planning to travel around to different points, work out the logistics, and write out a schedule to carry with you.

Be sure that you have new camera batteries and plenty of film. There's nothing worse than missing that irretrievable magic moment.

Carry emergency supplies for your friend, such as Vaseline, a dry T-shirt, spare socks, and a spare shoelace. Having such supplies could make you a marathon-day hero. Remember to pack food for yourself, too—you may not be in an area where food is accessible when you're hungry. And don't forget your money; virtually nothing is free in New York City.

An all-day "Fun Pass" MetroCard, for only $4, will give you unlimited rides on public transportation—subways *and* buses! (Using the subway system is far preferable to attempting to drive around the course in a car, as many roads will be closed to traffic.)

How to Spot Your Runner

It can be a nightmare trying to spot an individual in a field of 30,000 runners. Don't worry, though; after 16 miles, the runners are beginning to spread out. Here are a few helpful hints.

- Make sure you know exactly what the runner will be wearing and what the runner's bib number is.

- Scout the course before the day of the race, and decide whether you'll want to be on the left or right side of the road.

- Work out approximately what time the runner will be passing your viewing point.

■ Take advantage of the cell phone split-finder system, which allows you to track a runner en route.

■ Wear distinctive clothing, and make sure your runner knows what you will be wearing.

■ As soon as you can spot your runner, scream his or her name as loud as you can! The recommended area to assist your runner is at the 20-mile point—the crowd is traditionally rather sparse. Forget trying to assist between 16 and 18 miles—the dense and vocal crowds make it near-impossible.

■ Consider taking along a pair of binoculars to scout the road ahead.

Spectating, By Borough (In Brief)

Staten Island
Starting time: 11:15 A.M.

Although the start is spectacular, it's not a good idea to try to watch it. It will be well-nigh impossible to spot any friends; it's difficult to get to the starting area if you're a non-runner, and the corrals (into which the runners are shepherded before the start) are not accessible to you.

Runners must not only get through five boroughs but also over five bridges.

Bridge	Boroughs	Location
1. Verrazano-Narrows	Staten Island—Brooklyn	Miles 0–2
2. Pulaski	Brooklyn—Queens	Miles 13–13.5
3. Queensboro	Queens—Manhattan	Miles 15–16
4. Willis Avenue	Manhattan—Bronx	Miles 20–20.2
5. Madison Avenue	Bronx—Manhattan	Miles 21–21.2

And after the race starts, you'll be stuck for a considerable time in Staten Island. Better to go straight to Brooklyn.

At about 11:25 A.M. the lead runners will be across the Verrazano-Narrows Bridge and into Bay Ridge, Brooklyn.

Brooklyn

Of the five boroughs, Brooklyn enjoys the most mileage of the marathon. There are some excellent points from which to view the excitement of the race, with lots of fun as the locals bring the party to the street. Musicians and bands greet the runners throughout the borough. A great viewing area is around the 8-mile mark, where the women's and men's fields merge.

Queens

Approximate arrival of the race leaders: 12:15 P.M.

The runners are only in the borough of Queens for a short spell. Not a good borough for spectating.

Manhattan

Approximate arrival of the race leaders: 12:25 P.M.

Strongly recommended from Mile 16 to Mile 18 on First Avenue— probably the loudest cheering on the course.

Bronx

Approximate arrival of the race leaders: 12:52 P.M.

Rather sparse crowds, and the race spends only about one mile in this borough. Still, there are excellent chances of being able to assist your runner here with a cheer of encouragement or a drink.

Return to Manhattan

Approximate arrival of the race leaders: 12:57 P.M.

The leaders are back in the borough of Manhattan after about five minutes in the Bronx. The viewing spots are best where the course reenters the Upper East Side, from 96th Street and Fifth Avenue onward to the south.

Runners' Timetable

Mile	Male Leaders*	6 min./mile	8 min./mile	10 min./mile	12 min./mile
Verrazano-Narrows Bridge midpoint					
1 mile	11:19:52	11:21	11:23	11:25	11:27
Exiting the bridge at 92nd St.					
2 miles	11:24:44	11:27	11:31	11:35	11:39
4th Ave. & 83rd St.					
3 miles	11:29:36	11:33	11:39	11:45	11:51
4th Ave. & 64th St.					
4 miles	11:34:28	11:39	11:47	11:55	12:03
4th Ave. & 44th St.					
5 miles	11:39:20	11:45	11:55	12:05	12:15
4th Ave. & 23rd St.					
6 miles	11:44:12	11:51	12:03	12:15	12:27
4th Ave. & 5th St.					
7 miles	11:49:04	11:57	12:11	12:25	12:39
Flatbush Ave. & Ashland Place					
8 miles	11:53:56	12:05	12:19	12:35	12:51
Classon Ave. (off Lafayette)					
9 miles	11:58:48	12:11	12:27	12:45	1:03
Bedford Ave. & Lynch St.					
10 miles	12:03:40	12:07	12:35	12:55	1:15

*The race leaders' pace includes seconds, and has been set at a 2:07:43 marathon finishing pace, the current course record.

Mile	Male Leaders*	6 min./mile	8 min./mile	10 min./mile	12 min./mile
Bedford Ave. & South 3rd St.					
11 miles	12:08:32	12:23	12:43	1:05	1:27
Manhattan Ave.					
12 miles	12:13:34	12:29	12:51	1:15	1:39
Pulaski Bridge, southern end					
13 miles	12:18:16	12:35	12:59	1:25	1:51
Pulaski Bridge, nearly at the crest					
13.1 miles	12:18:45	12:30	12:59	1:26	1:52
Vernon Blvd. & 45th Ave.					
14 miles	12:23:08	12:41	1:07	1:35	2:03
Queensboro Bridge, eastern end					
15 miles	12:28:00	12:47	1:15	1:45	2:15
Queensboro Bridge, western end (entering Manhattan)					
16 miles	12:32:52	12:53	1:23	1:55	2:27
1st Ave. & 75th St.					
17 miles	12:37:44	12:59	1:31	2:05	2:39
1st Ave. & 95th St.					
18 miles	12:42:36	1:05	1:39	2:15	2:51
1st Ave. & 115th St.					
19 miles	12:47:28	1:11	1:47	2:25	3:03
Willis Ave. Bridge					
20 miles	12:52:20	1:17	1:55	2:35	3:15
Madison Ave. & 138th St.					
21 miles	12:57:12	1:23	2:03	2:55	3:27

Mile	Male Leaders*	6 min./mile	8 min./mile	10 min./mile	12 min./mile
5th Ave. & 120th St.					
22 miles	1:02:04	1:29	2:11	2:55	3:39
5th Ave. & 102nd St.					
23 miles	1:06:56	1:35	2:19	3:05	3:51
Central Park, East Drive near 84th St.					
24 miles	1:11:48	1:41	2:27	3:15	4:03
Central Park, East Drive near 66th St.					
25 miles	1:16:40	1:47	2:35	3:25	4:15
Central Park, near W. 62nd St.					
26 miles	1:21:32	1:51	2:41	3:35	4:27
Central Park, near W. 67th St.					
26.2 miles	1:23:43	1:53	2:43	3:37	4:29

(All times are approximate, and should be used as guidelines. For the elite women's approximate arrival times, subtract 25 minutes from the times on the chart.)

INTERVIEW:
Tesfaye Jifar, Course Record-Holder

Tesfaye Jifar recorded his first international win at the 2001 NYC Marathon. His time of 2:07:43 was a new course record, beating Juma Ikangaa's 2:08:01 from 1989. Jifar was no stranger to the marathon; he holds the Ethiopian national record of 2:06:49. We caught up with him the day after he set the New York record.

Q: *Tesfaye, why did you consider the New York City Marathon?*
TJ: When I started running in Ethiopia, I had heard of New York's race.

Q: *Did you find the course difficult?*

TJ: No, the marathon is always a challenge. It was not difficult.

Q: *What did you think of the crowd support?*

TJ: I was very happy—the people cheered for me the whole way.

Q: *Will this marathon be a special memory for you?*

TJ: Yes, not only because it was my first win. I wanted to say sorry to the people of New York for the terrible disaster last September.

Q: *You have family in Boston. Could you see yourself moving over to America, too?*

TJ: My family is back home in Ethiopia. Also, Ethiopia is very good for training.

Q: *Will you be back to New York?*

TJ: New York is my favorite marathon now!

Q: *Have you done any fun things here in New York?*

TJ: New York is good for walking around! There is much to see here.

Joan Benoit Samuelson, on New York City

Joan Benoit Samuelson, the American record-holder for the marathon, is a regular visitor to New York. The 1984 Olympic Gold Medalist placed third in the 1988 New York City Marathon. She also ran a very respectable 4:37 for a seventh-place finish in the 1983 Fifth Avenue Mile, arguably the world's most prestigious road mile race. Joan says that when she's in New York, she loves to visit the museums, tries to see some shows on Broadway, and always eats out at the great restaurants in the city. "There is such a choice of good Italian here," she says. "You know what they say—'Eat Pasta, Run faster.'" We found Joan slipping out from the Ritz Carlton to buy herself a bag of H & H bagels.

Chapter Nine

The Race

Begin the race erring on the side of caution. Don't blast out and get frustrated by the masses. It may be impossible to hit your split time in the first mile. Instead, start thinking about your splits at Mile Two or Three, when running free should be possible. Run relaxed, and enjoy the experience. This is a journey through New York; take in the sights and the flavor of the event. Try to keep your pace as consistent as possible. Don't sprint from group to group, or accelerate to impress the crowd. Many a runner has "died" after First Avenue, where the magnitude of the support can send caution to the winds.

Remember to stick to your drinking plan. At the stations that offer sponges, wipe your quadriceps and face to remove the salty dried sweat. This will help your skin breathe more efficiently—very important on a hot day.

Since the first five-borough marathon in 1976, when Fred Lebow realized his dream of uniting the city with a marathon footrace, the New York City Marathon course has remained virtually the same. However, the 2001 introduction of the East 90th Street entrance to Central Park and various changes due to road work have altered the route slightly.

PRE-RACE TIPS

■ If possible, try to drive, or run, the last few miles of the course for familiarization.

■ Try to get extra sleep in the last week, and don't worry if you have problems sleeping the night before the race due to nerves; nobody sleeps very well that night. As long as you're rested, you'll be okay.

■ Eat familiar foods the last few days before the race.

■ Watch The Weather Channel to see what conditions to expect.

■ Remember to take your racing shoes with you on race day, if you're not wearing them to the start. (Don't laugh—it's happened.)

■ Put $20 of emergency money in a Ziploc bag and pin it to the inside of your shorts. If a crisis occurs, you'll be better equipped. (Even after finishing the event, you might have a minor crisis: a cup of coffee might be the most important thing in the world for you and you'll be prepared.) It's a good idea to add some toilet paper to this bag as well.

■ If it's cold, smear petroleum jelly on your legs for insulation.

■ If you're running for fun, try labelling a disposable camera with your address and the correct postage. Then you can take snapshots during the race and deposit the camera in a mailbox along the course if you get tired of carrying it or you run out of film.

■ The marathon is very much a mental event. Believe in yourself, and expect to feel rough—everyone does!

The Course, In Brief

Staten Island (Start)
The athlete's village is at Fort Wadsworth, where the marathon breakfast is served. You start the actual race at one of the three colored starting areas at the beginning of the Verazzano-Narrows Bridge, by the toll plaza. The main race begins at approximately 11:15 A.M. After the singing of the National Anthem, cannon sounds start the race.

The first mile is uphill, to the highest point on the marathon course, 274 feet above sea level. The Verazzano is the longest single-span suspension bridge in the United States, and has been in operation since 1964.

Brooklyn (1.5 miles)
In Brooklyn, New York's second-most populated borough with more than 4 million residents, you'll exit the Verrazano Bridge and pass Fort Hamilton, the former home of General Robert E. Lee. The route then turns onto Fourth Avenue, on which you'll run nearly five miles. At Mile 8, the race passes the Williamsburg Savings Tower, the tallest building in Brooklyn, which you will have been able to see for a number of miles. In Brooklyn you'll run through Italian, Spanish, Orthodox Jewish, and many more ethnic neighborhoods. Bands play loudly through the early miles, and the crowds are simply fantastic. At Mile 12, you'll go through Greenpoint, where Mae West grew up.

Queens (13 miles)
When you cross the Pulaski Bridge, you'll be in Queens, the largest borough in the area. This is also the halfway point in the race. A prize is awarded by the Polish government to the first male and female runners to reach the bridge—if they go on to finish the race.

Aesthetically, this is not one of the race's nicer areas—it's mostly

"You could literally feel the sound. It brought me out in goose bumps, it surged through my veins like a flash fire, it took me straight to the verge of tears and beyond."

—Andy Blackford waxing lyrical *in Runner's World* magazine about running onto First Avenue at Mile 16

industrial. You'll leave Queens by running over the Queensborough Bridge.

The Queensborough Bridge (15 miles)

Former New York residents Paul Simon and Art Garfunkel once sang about this "feelin' groovy" bridge. There are no spectators at this point, and the uphill eastern half of the bridge takes quite an effort. However, when you exit the bridge down a curving ramp, you come to a real high point—Manhattan's First Avenue. The crescendo of noise can be heard for many blocks, and as you run right through it onto First Avenue, the crowds, packed ten-deep, are truly deafening.

Manhattan (16 miles)

You'll run straight up First Avenue in Manhattan for about four miles. The crowd continues to give amazing vocal support right up to 92nd Street, where you'll leave First Avenue and cross the Willis Avenue Bridge, which spans the Harlem River, and enter the Bronx. This is the dreaded 20-mile point, where many runners report hitting the "wall."

The Bronx (20 miles)

The Bronx is the only borough of New York City that is actually part of the mainland United States. The Bronx portion of the course is very small—just a one-mile visit to the fifth borough.

Return to Manhattan (21 miles)

You'll cross the Madison Avenue Bridge and reenter Manhattan. As you cross this bridge, you can see the famous Yankee Stadium on the right—home of the winningest team in baseball history.

The Harlem section of the course is another relatively barren stretch for crowd support; however, at about Mile 22, you'll turn onto the famous Fifth Avenue. It is at this point that runners can truly feel they are heading to the finish. Just before entering Central Park, you'll be able to see the white stone spiral of the Guggenheim Museum, designed by architect Frank Lloyd Wright, on your left. Just before you reach it, though, you'll take a turn at East 90th Street into Central Park, just before the 24-mile mark.

The crowds are dense from 100th Street and Fifth Avenue all the way to the finish line—but the park section is tough; the undulations are unwelcome to tired legs.

At 24 miles, the course passes behind the Metropolitan Museum of Art. This, one of the world's largest and most comprehensive art museums, marks a rolling section of the course that will continue past the 25th mile.

The Finishing Stretch (Final mile)

After exiting the park at East 60th Street, the race runs along Central Park South before turning back into the park at Columbus Circle. The last quarter-mile is uphill, but the crowd support and the sight of the world's most famous finish line make the climb easy. (Many finishers claim that they didn't notice the hill!)

Finish Line!

It feels great to stop! Be sure to smile for the cameras when you cross the line. (And if you'd like to receive one of the official finish-line photograph proofs for print-ordering purposes, don't stop your wrist stopwatch while crossing the line, as this may obscure your race number from the camera's view, making identification difficult. At the start of the finish chute, your ChampionChip is removed, and you are presented with a finisher's medal. Your Mylar blanket, water, and a food bag are all waiting for you. Next, you walk along a row of buses until you reach yours, and you collect your baggage. Then you move on to the Family Reunion Area to meet your family and/or friends. It usually takes about twenty minutes to get there after finishing the race.

Family Reunion

If you have a red number, your assigned area is between 73rd and 77th streets. You'll exit the park at 77th. If your number is green, your area is between 77th and 81st streets; you'll exit at 81st. If you've got a blue number, your area is between 81st and 85th; you'll exit at 85th. Pink and yellow numbers, have a fun reunion at the West 72nd Street Transverse in Central Park.

PROFILE
Alberto Salazar

"The city of New York made me," remembers the three-time NYCM winner. The legendary Salazar, who set a world record for the marathon distance during the 1981 race, loves to run in Central Park. What about eating in New York? "Mama Leone's—I have many happy memories from that restaurant." And entertaining? "I always like going to sporting events at Madison Square Garden." Of course, Alberto has many happy sporting memories of his own from New York City. His all-time favorite memory? "The 1981 race, when I set the record."

The Course, in Detail

Mile 1   Staten Island, uphill to the crest of the Verrazano-Narrows Bridge.

Mile 2   Fort Hamilton. This is a fast, downhill mile as the course exits the bridge.

Mile 3   Onto Fourth Avenue—a flat stretch of the course, through an area known for its Scandinavian immigrants.

Mile 4 Fourth Avenue continues. You reach the first water station.

Mile 5 St. Michael's Roman Catholic Church. The course stays straight and flat along Fourth Avenue.

Mile 6 Fourth Avenue. Coming up to the 10K split, you're passing through diverse ethnic neighborhoods—from African to Ukrainian.

Mile 7 Still flat on Fourth. You pass Washington Park, the home of the old Brooklyn Dodgers baseball team.

Mile 8 It is here that the men's and women's courses converge, at the 512-foot-tall Williamsburg Savings Bank.

Mile 9 Bedford-Stuyvesant is the largest African-American community in New York. The course takes a slightly uphill right turn off Fourth Avenue, but stays generally flat.

Mile 10 The course meanders a little here; the long, straight avenues are replaced by a series of turns.

Mile 11 The course passes through Williamsburg, a district known for its large Hasidic Jewish community. In the race's early days, marathoners reported near-silence from unprepared crowds in Williamsburg, but today the cheers are as loud as on Fourth Avenue.

Mile 12 You pass through Greenpoint, a Polish community that was a shipbuilding center in the 19th century. The marathon course is about to leave Brooklyn, and for the next few miles the terrain takes in a few undulations.

Mile 13 The Pulaski Bridge is a short, sharp surprise to the legs. The halfway point greets the runners with a slight challenge. Thankfully, the climb is brief.

Mile 14 Queens feels rather desolate in this industrial area, and again the course snakes through the streets. You're soon to pass Silvercup Studios, a former bakery that is now one of NYC's largest film studios. The popular TV show *Sex in the City* is produced here.

Mile 15 Hill work! The arduous incline up the Queensborough Bridge is a wake-up call to the muscles, and you still have a long way to go. There are no spectators here, and nobody seems to find this bridge easy. It's almost three-quarters of a mile of steady climbing, and then you crest the bridge and begin the long downhill slope into Manhattan.

Mile 16 A swing to the left off the ramp, and the runners, not unlike gladiators, arrive on First Avenue to a tumultuous roar. Truly a highlight of this marathon. You are now entering Yorkville, so named after the Duke of York, who sent ships to capture the city from the Dutch in the 17th century.

Mile 17 First Avenue is straight and flat, and the crowd's excitement has been known to entice runners to forget their game plans and speed up. There's still a long way to go. Feed off the energy, but beware, or even the slight undulations will take their toll.

Mile 18 A traditional point for tactical breaks at the front of the race. Tegla Loroupe started her attacks here; Grete Waitz also took command at this point in her first New York City Marathon. The road slopes downward, and the legs usually still feel fresh enough to take advantage of it.

Mile 19 The crowds thin out at this point, and you have a tough mile or two ahead. At least you're running on a flat part of this seemingly never-ending avenue.

Mile 20 The law of marathoning says that the second half of the marathon really begins at 20 miles. Sure, you only have 6 miles to go, but they are equally as challenging, if not more so, than the first 20! It is here that the body hits the infamous "wall" if your pace has been too fast, or your training incomplete. Now the true challenge of the marathon starts: a battle of the mind over the weary body.

To make matters worse, there's an ill-placed bridge to climb as the course enters the Bronx. The Willis Avenue Bridge is small, but at this point it feels harder to run than the Verrazano-Narrows Bridge in the first mile. A carpet gives the runners a reprieve from the iron grid underfoot. This mile twists and turns over a rolling terrain.

Mile 21   Onto Fifth Avenue, and luckily the course flattens out again. You'll get the feeling of truly heading home, and the crowd support starts to pick up through this Harlem neighborhood as you reenter Manhattan.

Mile 22   A couple of small turns take you around Marcus Garvey Park, and Central Park looms ahead, the trees to the right luminous as beacons. Central Park means that the finish line isn't far away. However, after 22 miles, the gentle uphill climb up Fifth Avenue feels like a mountain.

Mile 23   Runners used to enter the park here at 102nd Street. Nowadays the course continues up Fifth Avenue. A few wry smiles from veteran competitors were seen in 2001 when the organizers announced, "We have taken out the hill." Well, the new route up to East 90th Street remains very much a hill! It just stretches over a longer distance.

In the knowledge that the course will soon take a right turn into the park keeps most runners in motion.

Mile 24   Running in Central Park is invigorating, and you reach it at just the right time for a pick-me-up. Enthusiastic, buoyant crowds cheer the race through a section of the course that's far from flat. A long downhill to the Boathouse hammers the quadriceps, only to be followed by a short, rather steep uphill, which again at this stage feels like climbing the Empire State Building. The road twists for the next half mile, but the worst of the undulations are now over.

Mile 25   Another downhill, this time for a good quarter of a mile, greets the runners. For those with tired legs, this is not as welcome a sight as one might expect; downhills add shock and can hurt. You now exit the park and make a right turn onto Central Park South—a straight and slightly uphill half-mile, but knowing that you're so close does wonders for the legs.

At the end of Central Park South, the race swings to the right around

Columbus Circle. From here on, the crowds scream and yell, making each and every finisher feel like a champion.

Mile 26 The final 385 yards to the finish line adds a final sting—it's uphill!—but the crowds, the excitement, and the drama of finishing all smooth this incline out: The sense of achievement is overwhelming.

The Sweep Bus

Buses will follow the route, at approximately 15-minute-per-mile pace, to pick up runners who are not able to complete the course.

The Weather

New York State is not known for a stable climate, and the extremities can be very unhelpful to the marathon runner. Several times, most of them in the early days when the race was run in September and October, the heat and humidity have slowed the runners to a crawl. On other race days, the pouring rain and cold have nearly frozen the muscles of the athletes.

For variety, take 1992 and 1993. Runners complained about the cold in 1992, the next year they griped about the scorching heat!

In 1974, the humidity rose to 93 percent, and the heat caused a 40-percent dropout rate! Consider that in 1986, in temperate conditions, fewer than 100 runners dropped out from a field of 20,502.

Experiment with your race clothing in your long runs leading up to the marathon. The last 100 years of New

Irish-Canadian Peter Maher twice finished in the top ten at the NYC Marathon. His words of wisdom:

"My advice for first-timers:

1. Plan for all types of weather. This is very important in New York.
2. Be very careful in the transition from the uphill first mile to the downhill second mile—a great place to pull a hamstring. I tweaked mine badly there in 1990.
3. Just get to Central Park, 'cause the crowds from there home won't let you quit. I had a ringing in my head for hours after each time I ran the New York City Marathon."

York Novembers have never had temperatures below 30° F or above 83° F, so the odds are very good that these are your predictable extremes. Normally (see below), the weather is quite suitable to marathon running.

The average temperatures for the twenty-five years of NYC Marathon race-days are as follows:

Maximum	57° F/14° C
Minimum	43° F/ 6° C
Mean average	50° F/10° C

Mylar Blankets

A common sight near the finish line is runners wandering around looking like space cadets wrapped in silver heat-retaining blankets. These lightweight blankets are very effective—they really help keep your body temperature from plummeting after you've stopped running.

There are Mylar blankets not only at the finish but at each mile marker after Mile 3.

Undulation Profile

Comparatively, New York's course isn't too difficult. Although the race doesn't have a reputation of being lightning-fast (read "flat"), neither is it extremely demanding. Marathons such as Berlin, Chicago, and Rotterdam have carved their niches in history by being flat enough to allow top runners to challenge world-best times. New York, though, will almost certainly never see a world's best time set in its marathon. Should anyone care? What New York loses in speed it

> **"New York is the best marathon in the world, no question—just run it!"**
>
> —Pieter Langerhorst, manager of the Kenyan High Altitude Camp, and husband/coach of world-class marathoner Lornah Kiplagat

> "Don't worry about the hills; they aren't that bad. Last year, I was running with caution. This year, when I ran strongly, I won."
>
> —Rodgers Rop, men's champion, 2002

gains in spirit, character, and eminence as *the* premier marathon to run.

The hilliest part of the race is actually the first two miles. The first mile is uphill, and the second down, over the Verrazano-Narrows Bridge. Thus you can relax after the first mile, knowing that you're already over the biggest climb! The course flattens out considerably for the next ten miles. There's a short climb up the Pulaski Bridge, and then two miles later the much longer drag up the Queensboro Bridge. (At this point, you'd do well to focus on the upcoming energy of First Avenue—ample reward for the climb.) First Avenue is basically flat with a few gentle undulations. The small Willis Avenue Bridge at the 20-mile mark in the Bronx feels tough only because of the mounting fatigue. Running down Fifth Avenue from 102nd Street to Central Park's entrance at East 90th Street feels tough for the same reason; the actual elevation change is minimal.

Just before Mile 25 there's a sharp downhill followed by a short steep uphill that's hard on the quads, but you're nearly at the finish; take heart!

And yes, the last quarter-mile is also uphill, but hey, what better way to finish than on a high?

Having a friend on the course is an ace in the hole. If at all possible, persuade, bribe, or otherwise cajole someone to be out on the course for you between the 20th and 22nd miles.

Some useful items for your friend to bring: Gatorade, chocolate, flask of a favorite hot drink, spare socks, dry T-shirt, sandals, money, Aleve, replacement drinks, and sympathy!

Fluid Stations in the Marathon

The human body is about 60 percent water, and this underlines the importance of proper hydration. Running a marathon dehydrates the body faster than it is possible to rehydrate it, so it's vital to drink at the fluid stations.

Some common questions on hydration

Q: *In general, how much water should I aim to drink?*

A: A normal runner training in a mild climate should try to drink a minimum of 72 ounces per day.

Q: *Which is the better choice—a sports drink, or plain water?*

A: Plain water is absorbed much faster into the body, making it an excellent choice for the marathon.

Q: *How much water should I drink in the morning, of the race?*

A: As soon as you get up drink about 20 ounces of water slowly. Then drink your usual morning beverage—coffee, tea, whatever your routine dictates.

Continue to sip water until ninety minutes before the start of the race. Don't drink too much after that; it's not a good idea to start the race with your stomach too bloated. About twenty minutes before the starting gun, drink one last cup of water.

Q: *Is there water at the starting line?*

A: Yes, at Fort Wadsworth there will be plenty of water. However, consider taking your own bottle with you for safety's sake. That way if you're rushed and have to go straight to the starting corral, water won't be a worry.

Q: *When is the first water station on the course?*

A: The first station will be at Mile 3. There will be long lines of tables on both sides of the road. Thereafter, there will be a fluid station every single mile all the way to the finish.

Q: *Should I drink at every station?*

A: Not necessarily. A good system is to drink a small amount every twenty minutes. Don't try to drink too much; a little is often better for the stomach. If you run ten-minute miles, drink every two miles; five-minute miles, drink every four miles.

Q: *Is it best to drink while I'm running, or to stop and drink?*

A: It's a good idea to slow down as you approach the water station (watch out—there's often a congestion of runners), take a cup, come to a complete stop to drink carefully, and then resume running. Many faster runners do drink on the run, but it's hard to do without spilling a lot of what you've grabbed—it takes practice. Those who do try to drink while running often merely splash their faces with water and swallow nothing but air. Bill Rodgers came to a complete stop for each drink (and once more to tie a shoelace) while running a 2:09 marathon on the demanding Boston course!

Q: *Is it just water at the stations in New York?*

A: No, Gatorade is also offered. The Gatorade will be in green cups and on the first few tables at each station; the water will be on the later tables. The volunteers will shout out either "Gatorade" or "Water," making the distinction very clear to the runners.

Q: *I have tried to drink in training, and it feels awkward. Can I skip drinking?*

A: Tumo Turbo, an elite Ethiopian marathoner, never likes to drink during the race. However, in the drug-testing tent he is often the first athlete able to provide a urine sample! Turbo spends only a little over two hours on the roads, and he's an exception even among people his speed. Drink! If drinking feels unnatural, come to a complete stop and slowly sip half a cup of water. Carefully toss the cup in one of the trash cans provided and resume running.

Q: *Are there any special precautions one should take at a fluid station?*

A: Remember that as you're stopping or slowing, another runner may be accelerating away from the table. Be considerate and observant of those around you. Also, if you're wearing gloves, remove the glove from the hand that will take the cup, as if the glove gets wet it will stay that way for the entire race.

Q: *I want to practice drinking on the run. How can I do this?*

A: There are a number of ways. World Championship Marathon bronze medalist Steve Spence used to set up a table at his local running track and practice scooping up his bottle from the table and running with it while drinking. Other runners enter low-key races to learn the art. The simplest way is to carry a water-belt on your training runs. This is very smart if you're training in hot/ humid conditions.

> "When I came to New York in 1978, I was a full-time school teacher and track runner, and determined to retire from competitive running. But winning the New York City Marathon kept me running for another decade.
>
> —Grete Waitz, nine-time winner, New York City Marathon

The runners in New York's Central Park are lucky—water fountains can be found in abundance throughout the park. The NYRR organize special pre-marathon training runs that include drink tables for the participants.

If worse comes to worst, either plead with a friend to cycle with you on a training run, or drive your course before your run and hide water bottles along the route.

The water stations in the race can be rather intimidating. Often the first table is far too crowded, there are puddles of spilled water, and runners continually bump each other. A Swedish runner, Marielle Westlund, prefers to wear a belt with her own small bottles during the race. This way, she can avoid the pushing and shoving of the first few stations and rely on the fluid stations only in the later stages, when the field has strung out.

The elite runners have an advantage at the drinks stations: The top-seeded runners are allowed to place their own water bottles on a special table. They decorate their bottles to make them easy to spot, and often the liquid is a specially prepared "secret" drink to power them to the finish. (Frank Shorter was known to drink defizzed Coke, which gave him a caffeine boost; Moses Tanui prefers just plain water.) Although this is a huge benefit, there can be slip-ups. In the 1997 Rome Marathon, a Kenyan runner in the lead pack sprinted ahead at the midway point and grabbed a tall black bottle from the elite table. Moments later, Eddy Hellebuyck, an Olympian and American Masters record-holder, shouted out, "That's my (expletive) bottle!" A chase ensued!

Sponge Station
Between miles 18 and 19, on First Avenue, 30,000 water-soaked sponges are on hand for cooling and wiping the body.

Chapter Ten

After the Marathon

Recovery

After the marathon, it's important not to neglect your body's needs. Running 26.2 miles is a long and arduous task. Here are some tips for how to survive the following week and make the experience more enjoyable.

- Try not to stop dead in your tracks and sit down. This is the quickest way to get what experienced marathoners call Runner's Rigor Mortis. After receiving your finisher's medal, keep walking to the area where you'll collect your baggage. Get dressed (take off those soaked race clothes, if possible) and try to walk for another ten to fifteen minutes. This will really help to keep the blood flowing and wash the lactic acid and other waste products out of the muscles.

- Eat like an elephant. Whatever you have a hankering for, set about trying to find and eat it. Stefan Fridgeirsson of Iceland says, "I go straight to a hamburger restaurant and eat a few hamburgers. This is strange, as it is the only time I will eat hamburgers the

"After I won, it was time to celebrate. I had done a lot of running for this race and I was so relieved that it was all over. First I went out to a nice restaurant and had a steak and red wine, then the next day I went down Fifth Avenue to the shops, spending money on clothes for myself and presents for my children."

—Ludmila Petrova, women's champion, 2000

whole year!" Trust your body; it will tell you what it needs. Just make sure you eat as soon as possible to begin the process of rebuilding the damaged muscle tissue.

■ Drink water—it's the best way to rehydrate. Drink at least 32 ounces if possible. Stay away from carbonated and alcoholic drinks for the time being— neither can hydrate the body as quickly as water can, and hydration is the game plan.

■ If you have any really sore parts, try to get an ice pack on the area(s). If you're staying in a hotel, simply fill a plastic bag with cubes from an ice machine and apply it to the tender area for ten to fifteen minutes, then wait at least an hour, and repeat the cycle as many times as is convenient. This should reduce swelling and inflammation.

■ Pop an antiinflammatory pill, like Aleve or an ibuprofen product, with an additional glass of water.

■ If possible, soak in a lukewarm bath. (Cold water is even better, but after what you've just been through, we won't force you into an ice bath.)

■ Head for the bed. Take a couple of hours with the weight off your feet. Even if you can't sleep, watch a good movie and continue to drink and eat.

■ In the evening, head out to the Marathon Celebration Party, and try to walk for at least another ten minutes.

■ Some runners take a massage straight after the race. Hugh Jones, a London Marathon winner and 2:09 marathoner, goes looking for such treatment. Others prefer to wait a couple of days for the tissue to recover from the trauma of 26.2 miles of pounding before being kneaded and prodded.

The next day

■ Again, head for the water therapy; take a lukewarm bath or a warm shower.

■ If you have any pains or injuries, continue to ice the afflicted areas for ten- to fifteen-minute periods.

■ A twenty-minute walk is recommended, perhaps on a self-rewarding shopping spree.

■ Try to gently stretch the major muscle groups (quads, hamstrings, and calves) for ten minutes.

■ Eating is also a key factor of marathon recovery. Just as you tried to eat extra carbohydrates to go the distance, now is the time to eat extra to replenish the depleted stores. Overeat a bit—treat yourself to New York's great dessert cafes. (*See* Dining, pp. 138). However, try not to party past your normal sleeping hour; sleep is recovery's best friend.

■ Runners typically cross the finish line and say, "Never again." Five minutes later, they're planning their next marathons. A word of warning: Most successful marathon runners run no more than two marathon races per year. Give yourself a break from the training and pounding. By all means resume running, after a break of a week or so, but don't go straight back into a marathon training program. Reward your body, and stay away from runs of over forty minutes. The New York

> "After running the marathon, my legs are fine—only my face muscles are tired from smiling so much."
>
> —Joyce Chepchumba,
> women's champion, 2002

Marathon would complement running a spring marathon, such as London, Paris, Boston, or Cleveland.

Dining After the Marathon

After finishing the race, many athletes are left with a "now what?" feeling. You've put so many months of work into this one day; it's a good idea to plan a post-race celebration. The Marathon Celebration Party on the evening after the race is an excellent place to dance (easy!), swap marathon stories, and watch the award winners collect the hardware. In the days following the race, if you're lucky enough to be able to extend your NYC visit, you can choose one of these café/restaurants to really treat yourself!

Here's a concise list of "close to the finish line" indulgence eateries:

Upper East Side

Lenox

1278 3rd Avenue

(212) 772-0404

The ambiance of the quaint Upper East Side, and luxurious food at affordable prices.

Delectable Desserts

Payard's Pâtisserie

1032 Lexington Avenue (between 73rd and 74th streets)

(212) 717-5252

The cream of the crop; if a sweet reward is what you savor, no place is better than here.

Upper West Side

Café Mozart

154 West 70th Street

(212) 595-9797

A café dedicated to serving the finest cakes and desserts, set in a casual surrounding with live music. A huge array of delicious cakes, such as the name-deserving Moon Mountain Torte, makes this an ideal post-race celebration spot.

Café Lalo
201 West 83rd Street
(212) 496-6031
Of *You've Got Mail* fame. Great desserts at reasonable prices.

Columbus Bakery
474 Columbus Avenue
(212) 724-6880
Very close to where the runners exit Central Park after completing the marathon, this café's wide array of scrumptious pastries at moderate prices makes it an ideal post-race rendezvous.

Edgar's Café
255 West 84th Street
(212) 496-6126
Nice relaxing atmosphere with marathon-sized dessert awards.

Serendipity
38 East 58th Street
(212) 838-3531
A family-friendly mid-priced hot spot famed for its desserts.

Manhattan Sports Bars
Blondies
212 West 79th Street
New York, NY 10124
(212) 362-4360

No Idea
30 East 20th Street
New York, NY 10003
(212) 777-0100

Mustang Sally's Saloon
324 7th Avenue
New York, NY 10001
(212) 695-3806

ESPN Zone
1472 Broadway
New York, NY 10036
(212) 921-3776

Time Out
349 Amsterdam Avenue
New York, NY 10024
(212) 362-5400

ATHLETE PROFILE

Grete Waitz, Nine-Time NYC Marathon Champion

Q: *What three pieces of advice would you give to a New York first-timer?*

GW: New York is not an easy course—very few runners set PRs in that marathon. So be reasonable when you're aiming for a certain time.

Be prepared to spend a long time at the starting area. Bring extra clothes, food, and drink.

And don't get carried away in the first half. Save energy for the second half, which is a lot harder.

Q: *What, if any, are your enduring memories of your first win?*

GW: The marathon in '78 was my first road race. I had not run longer than 11 miles or so. I was in pain—a different kind of pain than I'd experienced running track—over the last four or five miles, and I promised myself I would never do this again.

> **COMMITMENT!**
>
> "Even in the worst weather, Fred Lebow was at all the New York races. He'd be standing there in the rain, soaked, greeting runners at the finish line. You felt an obligation to Fred, knowing he'd always be there."
>
> —NYC runner Blair Boyer, remembering the man behind the New York City Marathon

I remember being awestruck when we came to the starting area and saw so many people, and many of them didn't look like runners. Not the way I was used to seeing in Europe.

The first part felt soooo easy, and I thought marathon running was easy—until everything changed almost within a block.

I loved the crowds. I had never experienced anything like that earlier in my running career.

Q: *How does NYC differ from other races you have run?*

GW: The atmosphere, the excitement, all the runners from other countries, and the crowds make New York a very colorful and fun marathon to run. The crowds are so supportive of everybody out there. It doesn't matter if you're slow or fast, they make everybody feel like a winner. For the runners from abroad, it's also fun to be a part of the breakfast run on Saturday morning. The race is also very well organized. The NYRR does a fantastic job.

Q: *I heard about your special pre-race 1978 diet. Did you stay with this diet?*

GW: I really don't recommend that for anybody. In '78, "hydration" and "carbo-loading" were words I had never heard before. I had no idea how to prepare, nutrition-wise, for a marathon. But it proves that the most important element is the training and doing the miles—you can't eat or drink yourself to being a good runner.

Q: *Are there any fun things you always like to do when in New York?*
GW: When I'm in New York I just love walking the streets and watching the busy life and all the different people. Central Park on a Saturday or Sunday afternoon is great.

Q: *Do you have a favorite place in New York City that's non-running-related?*
GW: As an avid book enthusiast and audio-book listener, I love to spend time at Borders or Barnes and Noble.

Q: *Your name will be forever linked with the event. If you were to describe the New York City Marathon experience in one sentence, what would it be?*
GW: The New York City Marathon is a race you don't want to miss during your life as a runner.

Chapter Eleven

Things to Do and Places of Interest in New York

The International Friendship Run

The day before the marathon, at 8 A.M., more than 10,000 runners from more than 100 countries participate in this noncompetitive four-mile run from the United Nations building to Central Park, where they are treated to a complimentary breakfast.

The run is a wonderful sight. Runners wear or carry their countries' flags and colors, and many of them chant or sing songs as they run. If a four-mile run fits your schedule for the day before the race, this one's not to be missed. Many runners take the opportunity to trade T-shirts and pins from their countries following the run.

The annual presentation of the Abebe Bikila Award takes place before the start, honoring an individual who has made an outstanding contribution to the world of running.

Ronald McDonald House Kids' Half-Mile Fun Run

This is an event for the 8- to 18-year-olds. Kids have the chance to run across the finish line, and the $10 entry fee benefits Ronald McDonald House. It's held on the Saturday before the marathon, at 1 P.M.

For local high school runners, there's an invitational road race at 8:30 A.M.

New York Attractions

Bronx Zoo
2300 Southern Boulevard
Bronx, NY 10460
(718) 367-1010

Simply put, this is the largest and most extensive urban zoo in America. There's even a 6.5-acre African rainforest for the gorillas!

This attraction takes at least a day to appreciate, especially if you include such experiences as the camel ride. There is an interactive children's section of the zoo. Don't miss the lions and tigers, and consider boarding a Skyfari gondola that takes you above the park for an aerial view.

Cathedral of St. John the Divine
(212) 316-7540

The world's largest cathedral, St. John the Divine is located on Manhattan's Upper West Side at 112th Street and Amsterdam Avenue. It's open Monday through Saturday from 7 A.M. to 6 P.M. and Sunday from 7 A.M. to 8 P.M. The grounds and gardens are open during all daylight hours. Sitting in the gardens and listening to the church music is indeed a moving experience. Public tours take place Tuesday through

Saturday at 11 A.M. and Sunday at 1 P.M. The cost is $3.00, and the tour meets at the Visitor Center.

Central Park

59th Street and Fifth Avenue

Bordered by Central Park South (59th Street) Central Park West (Eighth Avenue), Central Park North (110th Street), and Fifth Avenue.

New York, NY 10019

(212) 310-6600

Manhattan's green pearl. Not only is this park a runner's paradise, but the grassland is a hub of entertainment. In New York, hardly a bad word is uttered about this sprawling 860-acre urban oasis. Architects Frederick Law Olmstead and Calvert Vaux took twenty years to design the park and supervise its construction. It was opened to the public in 1876 as "the people's park." Aside from the obvious sporting benefits (*all* the featured runners in this book called Central Park a great place to run), there are outdoor music concerts, free opera, and plays being performed throughout the summer and fall. Due to its huge expanse, this park has so many themes that one could easily spend a day riding the carousel, swimming for free in Lasker Pool, having a picnic lunch in Sheep Meadow, and eating an ice cream by the beautiful Bethesda Fountain. Each Sunday afternoon, you can listen to jazz at the northern end of the park. The options are endless, but here's a list of the park's main features:

- Baseball and softball fields
- Basketball courts
- Boat rentals
- Carousel
- Delacorte Theatre (Shakespeare in the Park)

■ Hiking trails

■ Ice-skating rink

■ Nature trails

■ Running trails galore (*see* Where to Run in NYC, page 63)

■ Restaurants

■ The Boathouse, Tavern on the Green

■ Picnic tables

■ Playgrounds

■ Ponds

■ Soccer fields

■ Tennis courts

■ Visitors' center

Central Park Wildlife Center and Zoo
830 Fifth Avenue
Central Park
New York, NY 10021
(212) 861-6031
Set in the heart of Manhattan, the Center offers the visitors the chance to see animals in environs close to their own. Sea lions and polar bears reside near domestic animals like cows and sheep. There is also an extensive aviary, and educational animal shows take place at the in-house Acorn Theater.

City Hall Park
Broadway and Chambers Street
Built two hundred years ago, City Hall has recently been renovated.

"This landmark building has been home to fifty-seven mayoral administrations and has been the seat of city government for 186 years," said then-Mayor Rudy Giuliani.

Chrysler Building
405 Lexington Avenue at 42nd Street

New York, New York 10174

(212) 682-3070

Snubbed by the Empire State Building after only a couple of months as the world's tallest skyscraper, this office building is among the best that the 1930s had to offer. Although there are no organized tours, the lobby, set in radiant chrome, is open daily to tourists.

Ellis Island and the Statue of Liberty
More than 40 percent of the U.S. population are descended from the 17 million immigrants that entered the United States through Ellis Island from 1892 to 1954. The Ellis Island Museum is housed in the exact building in which immigrants were processed during that time. Ferries leave from Manhattan's Battery Park, and there is the option of visiting the Statue of Liberty, located on nearby Liberty Island.

The famous statue was a gift from France. The trip to Liberty Island takes approximately fifteen minutes. Round-trip fare is $8 for adults, $6 for senior citizens, $3 for children ages 3–17, and free to children 3 and under. It's open seven days a week, from 9:30 A.M. to 5 P.M. For ferry schedules and information, call (212) 269-5755, or log on to *www.statueoflibertyferry.com*

Empire State Building
350 5th Avenue

New York, NY 10118

(212) 736-3100

Who in the world hasn't heard of the Empire State Building? Certainly nobody who saw *Sleepless in Seattle*. On a clear day, a trip up the

102 floors gives one an incomparable vista over the city of New York and beyond. A must, if only for the "been there, done that" NYC experience.

Built in 1931, and at that time the world's tallest skyscraper, it is—regrettably—once again New York's tallest building.

The observatory is open seven days a week, 9:30 A.M. to midnight (last tickets sold at 11:25 P.M.). Special holiday hours are observed. Admission is $11 for adults, $9 for military personnel and senior citizens, $6 for children ages 5–11, and free for children under 5 and in military uniform. For security reasons, bring a picture ID.

Gracie Mansion
(212) 570-4751

Set in the Upper East Side of Manhattan near the water, the mayor's house is on East End Avenue and East 88th Street.

It was built in 1799 by Archibald Gracie, a Scottish emigrant and one of the wealthiest men in the city. Fiorello H. La Guardia moved into Gracie Mansion in 1942 with his family, and this inaugurated the building as the official residence of the mayor of New York.

Tours: by reservation, every Wednesday at 10 A.M., 11 A.M., 1 P.M., and 2 P.M.

Grand Central Terminal
(212) 340-2210

A nexus of movement and energy, overwhelming in its grandeur and intricacy. Well worth a visit for one of the free tours that show the construction, design, and history of this New York transportation hub. The tours are on Wednesday and Friday at 12:30 P.M., and on the weekends at 11 A.M. Call the hotline for details, or simply hop off the 4, 5, 6, 7, or S subway train at 42nd Street.

Grant's Tomb
122nd Street and Riverside Drive
(212) 666-1640

In the largest mausoleum in the United States, two-term U.S. President Ulysses S. Grant rests beside his wife. Free admission allows the visitor to view memorabilia from the life of the Civil War general seven days a week from 9 A.M. to 5 P.M. The architecture follows that of Napoleon's tomb in Paris and is modeled of imposing white granite.

Jacob K. Javits Center
11th Avenue between 34th and 39th streets
(212) 216-2000
Take the A, C, or E train to 34th Street and walk west three blocks.

Currently the site for the New York City Marathon's Exposition and number pick-up. Dubbed "The Marketplace for the World," the new and improved Javits Center offers interactive kiosks to check the latest news and send e-mail; television and Webcasting facilities; private office suites and workstations; and restaurants and snack shops.

Lincoln Center of Performing Arts
Broadway between 62nd and 63rd streets
(212) 875-5000

The hub of performance culture in New York City, this large complex is home to the world-famous Juilliard School of Music, Avery Fisher Hall, the Metropolitan Opera House, the New York State Theater, the Mitzi Newhouse Theater, the New York Public Library and Museum of the Performing Arts, and the Vivian Beaumont Theater. Take the 1 train to 66th Street/Lincoln Center.

Metropolitan Museum of Art
1000 Fifth Avenue
New York, NY 10028
(212) 535-7710

The huge and imposing classic nineteenth-century stone building on Fifth Avenue is the largest museum in the world. More than two million artifacts currently belong to the Met. At least one full day—and probably much longer—is needed to taste and enjoy the many splendors of this institution.

Museum of Modern Art
11 West 53rd Street
New York, NY 10019
(212) 708-9480

Founded in 1929, MoMA holds a staggering 100,000-plus works of art (sculptures, prints, film, photographs, and, of course, pictures). Literally a whole day should be put aside to fully explore these expanses of captured beauty. The museum was expanded in the 1980s, but weekends (when admission is a donation of your choice) find this building packed to the rafters.

NASDAQ MarketSite
43rd Street and Broadway

An interactive experience designed to illuminate the future of investing in the techno-world. Located in Times Square, MarketSite uses the latest technology to bring today's—and tomorrow's—stock market to life.

The hours are Monday through Thursday from 9 A.M. to 8 P.M., Friday from 9 A.M. to 10 P.M., Saturday from 10 A.M. to 10 P.M., and Sunday from 10 A.M. to 8 P.M. The entrance fee is $7.

Call 1-877-NASDAQ-1 (1-877-627-3271)

Take the N, R, S, 1, 2, 3, or 7 train to Times Square station.

New York Aquarium
Boardwalk at West 8th Street
Brooklyn, NY 11224
(718) 265-3474

Located at Coney Island, this is a pearl of a find for the ocean enthusiast. An aqua-theater lets us watch dolphins, sea lions, and walruses. A coastline and salt marsh have been built within a discovery cove. This is an unexpected and delightful place to explore the wonders of the sea.

New York Botanical Gardens
Bronx River Parkway at Fordham Road
Bronx, New York 10458
(718) 817-8700

One of the largest and oldest botanical gardens in the United States. It includes the Haupt Conservatory and walking trails throughout 250 acres, which also includes forty acres of New York City's original forest. A popular location for NYC weddings and receptions.

Take the D or the 4 train to Bedford Park, then take the #26 bus east. There is also a weekend shuttle from Manhattan by reservation.

New York Public Library
Fifth Avenue and 42nd Street
New York, New York 10018
(212) 930-0830

Another culture center in the heart of Manhattan. Bryant Park, to the west of the library, makes for an ideal reading setting with its relative inner-city peace. Throughout the summer months, a Monday-night film festival takes place in the park.

Free tours of the library take place Monday through Saturday at 11 A.M. and 2 P.M.

Hours: Monday and Thursday–Saturday from 10 A.M. to 6 P.M.; Tuesday and Wednesday from 11 A.M. to 7:30 P.M. Admission is free.

Take the 1, 2, 3, B, D, N, R, F, or Q train to 42nd Street, or the 7 train to Fifth Avenue.

Prospect Park Wildlife Center
450 Flatbush Avenue
Brooklyn, NY 11225
(718) 399-7339

Why not finish a run in Prospect Park with a tour of this educational animal center? Three exhibit areas highlight the world of animals: their lifestyles, and their places in our lives. There are more than eighty species of animals at the Center.

Queens Wildlife Center
53-51 111th Street
Queens, NY 11368
(718) 271-7761

Situated in Flushing Meadows. Visitors get the chance to see native North American animals that are now far from our everyday lives. You'll see bison, buffaloes, and mountain lions—and be sure to take in the open aviary.

Riverside Church
Riverside Drive and Claremont Avenue, between 120th and 122nd streets

Riverside Church is modeled after the 13th-century Gothic cathedral in Chartres, France. It opened in 1930. Open daily from 7 A.M. to 10 P.M.

Rockfeller Center
30 Rockfeller Plaza
Fifth to Sixth Avenues
New York, NY 10012
(212) 632-3975

A tourist site seen each morning as the *Today* show's street studio. A huge, underground twenty-four-acre shopping arcade with more than 300 shops, where almost everything and anything to do with New York can be found.

In November, Rockfeller Center is home to a giant imported Christmas tree.

Roosevelt Island Tramway
(212) 832-4540

Many tourists deem a four-minute tram-ride from Manhattan to Roosevelt Island too short. The *New York Times* raved about the ride as "the most exciting view in New York City!" Once you're on Roosevelt Island, the views of Manhattan's East Side are spectacular, and a 25-cent bus ride will take you to some serene picnic spots and a calm outside the storm of the city. Running around the perimeter of the island is a completely flat three miles.

The tramway leaves from Second Avenue and 60th Street on Sunday through Thursday from 6 A.M. to 2 A.M. and on Friday and Saturday until 3:30 A.M. and costs a mere $1.50 each way. Students with tram permits ride free; senior citizens and the disabled pay $1.50 round-trip.

Rye Playland
Playland Parkway
Rye, NY 10580
(914) 813-7010
Loads of rides and attractions ensure a great day out for the whole family. There are even an ice rink and a beach for diversity! All the rides and attractions require tickets (at 75 cents apiece, although many rides and attractions require more than one ticket) that can be purchased in booklets or individually.

Saint Patrick's Cathedral
Fifth Avenue at 50th Street
(212) 753-2261
Built in the classic French Gothic style in 1879, this cathedral is currently the 11th largest church in the world.

South Street Seaport
Fulton Street to the Brooklyn Bridge
Manhattan has it all, including a chance to view some restored eighteenth- and nineteenth-century buildings in what was once one of

the busiest seaports on the East Coast. A museum lets us see how the old seaport used to look.

Staten Island Ferry
Whitehall Terminal at Whitehall Street and South Street

(718) 815-BOAT

Perhaps the best bargain in New York. For what many consider the best views of the Statue of Liberty and the lower Manhattan skyline, take the free twenty-four-hour service that runs seven days a week. Phone for a time schedule.

Staten Island Zoo
614 Broadway

West Brighton

Staten Island, NY 10310

(718) 442-3100

Set in a beautiful nineteenth-century surround, this center is a gem on Staten Island. Recommended are its serpentarium, aquarium, and tropical forest display. However, if it's a large variety of animals you're after, it's better to stick to the Bronx.

Strawberry Fields
Near West 72nd Street in Central Park

New York, NY 10001

Almost all European visitors to New York want to go to Strawberry Fields, the memorial field for the late Beatle John Lennon. Just across the road from this area of Central Park is the famed Dakota building where John and his wife Yoko Ono lived until his untimely death on December 8, 1980. The 2.5-acre plot of land is a popular and peaceful place for picnics.

One block away is the San Remo building, where Lennon parked his multicolored Rolls Royce.

Theater District

42nd to 53rd streets, between Sixth and Eighth avenues

Amazingly, thirty-six major theaters are located here, hosting some of the world's most famous productions—all packed within this small strip of Manhattan. The theater ambiance is everywhere—watch the restaurant rush as the curtain call nears.

Theodore Roosevelt House

28 East 20th Street, between Park Avenue and Broadway

(212) 260-1616

This house is a reconstruction built in 1923, but it was here that President Roosevelt spent the first fourteen years of his life.

Open Wednesday through Sunday from 9 A.M. to 5 P.M. Tours every hour until 4 P.M. Admission is $2.

Times Square

42nd to 47th Streets along Broadway

New York, NY 10001

(212) 768-1560

Known as the crossroads of the world. Where the performing arts share equal billing with urban commerce. Visit Times Square at night for an electric energy that's hard to find elsewhere in the world. A dazzling array of neon lights, and electric advertising in all media illustrate the theme that New York City never sleeps. This is the site of the world's biggest New Year's Eve party, but at any time of year it's worth a visit if only to witness the diversity and individuality of this city. Sports fans should visit the ESPN Zone at 1472 Broadway and 42nd Street. Here you'll find a huge sports-entertainment complex with an American grill–style restaurant.

Trinity Church

Broadway at Wall Street

Built in 1697, Trinity Church

The average runner takes 3,000 steps per mile.

ranks as one of the oldest in the United States. Rebuilt twice, the last time in 1846, it is open Monday through Friday from 8:00 A.M. to 6 P.M. and weekends from 8 A.M. to 4 P.M. Guided tours, Monday through Friday at 2 P.M.

TV Shows

New York is the mecca of tabloid TV. If you want to stand in line for a few hours, the tickets are free to such shows as the *Today* show, *The Late Show with David Letterman*, *Late Night with Conan O'Brien*, and *Saturday Night Live*.

United Nations
First Avenue at 46th Street
(212) 963-7113

The only piece of land in Manhattan that is not part of the United States. The colorful 181 flags in front represent all of the member countries' undertaking to work together for a united world. Guided tours begin every fifteen minutes, from 9:15 A.M. to 4:45 P.M. Admission is $7.50 for adults, $6 for seniors, $5 for students, and $4 for kids ages 5–14. Children under 5 are not permitted on the tour. For tours in other languages, call (212) 963–7539. Reservations are required for groups of fifteen or more.

FIFTEEN TOURISTS' FAVORITE THINGS TO DO IN NYC

1. The Staten Island Ferry. It's a great way to see the city, and it's like being in the United Nations. People from around the world ride that thing.

—John Conley, Austin, Texas

2. The Empire State Building on a crisp clear morning. If it's cloudy, save it for another day.

—Jose Garcia, Madrid, Spain

3. A jet-boat ride round Manhattan. —Claudia Aquino, Minnesota

4. Central Park. Even if you're not a runner, there is so much to do and see there. The amazing contrast of greenery inside the urban sprawl is unique. The fall weather brings out all the beautiful colors. —Anders Szalkai, Stockholm, Sweden

5. We went to the Metropolitan Museum of Art at about five P.M. and looked at some of the exhibits; then we went to the balcony and ordered wine and bruschetta and listened to the quartet play classical music, all while surrounded by beautiful works of art. The museum is open until nine P.M., so we were able to walk around afterward and enjoy more of the exhibits and then cross the street to Melrose for dessert.
—Michael Maloney, Florida

6. Going to the Jekyll and Hyde bar. Drink beer from the yards [a glass holding a yard of ale]. I love the atmosphere of the small pub, with all the scientific laboratory artifacts. —Mike Mykytok, world-class runner, New Jersey

7. Going to Times Square in the evening, then enjoying a show.
—Natalie Armstrong, Belgium

8. Just to walk around and take it all in is my best advice. Enjoy the streets and the people. —Martin Armstrong, Belgium

9. Strolling down Fifth Avenue, window shopping in the posh shops.
—Bryndis Magnusdottir, Reykjavik, Iceland

10. Visit the best jazz clubs in the country. Even the small hole-in-the-walls, in the Village for example, have great acts that you've never heard of but probably will someday. The collection of talent, in all fields, is what makes New York such a great city.
—Philip Bentley, Eugene, Oregon

11. To enjoy a Cosmopolitan, some nice piano music, and great views of downtown Manhattan at the River Café cocktail bar right under the Brooklyn Bridge. Preferably outside, right next to the water, during a warm summer night.
—Anke Dieker, Munich, Germany

12. Dancing at the Swing 46 club. —Lars-Åke Johnson, Stockholm, Sweden

13. Shopping, and then cocktails in that high-up hotel!

—Shirley O'Shea, Cork, Ireland

14. Taking a bus tour of Manhattan.

—Rolf Olsen, Denmark

15. A horse-carriage ride in Central Park in the moonlight.

—Dave Courtney, Great Britain

ATHLETE PROFILE

John Kagwe, Two-Time NYC Marathon Champion

Q: *What do you like about New York?*

JK: It is a wonderful city, with very nice, encouraging people.

Q: *Obviously, winning the marathon here twice has made NYC special for you, but do you think you'd like New York as a city otherwise?*

JK: The marathon is difficult, you have to learn to run the race here. At first when I came I did not win, but each year I learned a little more. I like the city because the people cheer regardless of what country you come from.

Q: *What is your advice to any marathon runner attempting New York?*

JK: Don't do anything crazy until you are past the eighteen-mile mark, even if you feel good. The park is tough.

Q: *What do you do in New York City, apart from running, when you're here?*

JK: Nothing. I try to relax before the race. Maybe visit the Expo, but little else. It is an exciting city, so you must save energy for the race.

Q: *Do you train differently for New York than for other marathons?*

JK: Not really. There are no secrets to training for the marathon—just hard work. Each marathon becomes difficult unless you have done very good training; then it is not so hard!

Q: *Can you give us one example of a hard marathon training session for you?*

JK: In preparation I often run with runners who are preparing for shorter events, to sharpen my speed. Running long is not a problem for me, but to run fifteen times 400 meters in sixty or sixty-one seconds while running 120 miles per week is very tough, my legs are always tired. When I train for the marathon I like to go to bed feeling that my legs are finished, they have no more energy to give me—they can run no more for the day. That is marathon training.

Chapter Twelve

Facts and Figures

NEW YORK CITY MARATHON COURSE RECORD PROGRESSION

Women

2:55:22	Beth Bonner	USA	09/19/71
2:46:14	Kim Merritt	USA	09/28/75
2:39:11	Miki Gorman	USA	10/24/76
2:32:30*	Grete Waitz	NOR	10/22/78
2:27:33*	Grete Waitz	NOR	10/21/79
2:25:42*	Grete Waitz	NOR	10/26/80
2:25:29	Allison Roe	NZL	10/25/81
2:24:40	Lisa Ondieki	AUS	11/01/92
2:24:21	Margaret Okayo	KEN	11/04/01

Men

2:31:38	Gary Muhrcke	USA	09/13/70
2:22:54	Norman Higgins	USA	11/19/71
2:21:54	Tom Fleming	USA	09/30/73

*World Best performance

2:19:27	Tom Fleming	USA	09/28/75
2:10:10	Bill Rodgers	USA	10/24/76
2:09:41	Alberto Salazar	USA	10/26/80
2:08:13	Alberto Salazar	USA	10/25/81
2:08:01	Juma Ikangaa	TAN	11/05/89
2:07:43	Tesfaye Jifar	ETH	11/04/01

Masters' Course Records

2:30:17	Priscilla Welch	GBR	Aged 42, in 1987
2:14:34	John Campbell	NZL	Aged 41, in 1990

A Marathon of . . .

1,000 yellow marathon banners; 1.5 million cups of water; 800 plastic garbage cans; 218 buses making 297 trips (for runners and press); 13,700 NO PARKING signs; 2.5 tons of finishers' medals; 33 TV cameras; 300 gallons of marathon-blue road paint; 807 portable toilets; 76,000 finish photos; 11 helicopters; 346 finishers *per minute* at peak time; 100 massage therapists; 100,000 Aleve tablets; 70 million TV viewers; 2 million spectators; 75,000 visitors to the Expo; 2,828 New York police officers along the course; and 114 international flags!

Recognize That Face in the Park?

All these celebs and more are known to run in Central Park. Ralph Lauren (designer), Madonna (singer-actor), Howard Stern (radio personality), Paul McCartney (singer-songwriter), Darryl Hannah (actor), Christopher Walken (actor), Christian Slater (actor), Summer Sanders (Olympic medal winner, swimming; host of *NBA Inside Stuff*), Mike Malinin (drummer for the Goo Goo Dolls rock band).

And celebrities who have finished the marathon include model

Kim Alexis, world heavyweight champion boxer Ingemar Johanssen, rock star David Lee Roth, actress Mariel Hemingway, and ski champion Jean-Claude Killy.

Other New York City Races

New York is a premier running city, with typically more than one race per week. The author's top twelve picks are:

January: The Fred Lebow Classic 5-Miler, in Central Park. Run to honor the late, great Fred.

February: The Snowflake 4-miler, in Central Park. A classic road race that usually marks the start of serious NYC racing.

March: The Brooklyn Half-Marathon. The first time-trial for many who are thinking think about the year's upcoming marathon. Also the first in the NYRR's half-marathon series—one in each borough.

April: The Queens Half-Marathon. The tour of the boroughs continues with this two-loop race through residential Queens.

May: The Carey Wall Street 4.01K Rat Race. A theme race at its best. Run in the evening through the bustling financial district. First finishers in business attire, including briefcase, win awards. (And yes, the distance is 4.01K.)

June: New York's Mini Marathon. The world's best women runners come to the city and rule the streets of New York for a day in this women-only race, open to both elite and recreational runners. Site of the current women's world road record for 10K, set in 2002 by Morocco's Asmae Leghzaoui.

July: The Bronx Half-Marathon. Third stop on the half-marathon tour. By now marathon fever has hit the city, and it's time to get into training mode. This race is a wake-up call.

August: The Manhattan Half-Marathon. Borough number four—two loops of Central Park. How many big cities can boast a City-Center half-marathon with zero traffic on the road?

September: Van Cortlandt Park Cross-Country Races. A series of cross-country races is held in this beautiful parkland a few miles north of Manhattan.

October: The Staten Island Half Marathon. The half-marathon tour's final stop—with one month to go until the Big Day, this almost feels like a dress rehearsal.

November: The New York City Marathon. For me, the only marathon worth running!

December: The Hot Chocolate 15K. Hot chocolate and plenty of bagels are waiting at the finish line, making running really worthwhile!

For details on all the above races, check out the www.nyrrc.org Web site.

The Top Three Closest Winnings Margins

WOMEN

■ In 1990, Wanda Panfil of Poland defeated Kim Jones of the United States by a mere five seconds.

- Russia's Ludmila Petrova's victory in 2000 was only 18 seconds in front of fast-closing Franca Fiacconi of Italy.

- Anuta Catuna of Romania was ahead of Fiacconi by just 24 seconds in 1996. A relieved Catuna dedicated her win to the memory of Fred Lebow, the former race director.

MEN

- There was drama aplenty when German Silva and Benjamin Paredes, both Mexicans, were separated by only two seconds in 1994, after Silva had taken his wrong turn in the final mile.

- In 1998, defending champion John Kagwe coolly waited until the final 400 meters to kick away from his countryman Joseph Chebet, winning by just three seconds.

- American Alberto Salazar's third victory, in 1982, was his closest—a mere four seconds ahead of Mexico's Rodolfo Gomez.

Resources

New York City Running Clubs

Why not hook up with a local running team for a training run? Most local clubs welcome runners to join their groups for a pre-marathon workout. Call and ask for specific details:

Achilles Track Club
Manhattan based, for disabled runners
Contact: (212) 354-0300

Brooklyn Road Runners
Open club in Brooklyn
Contact: (718) 921-7183

Central Park Track Club
Manhattan-based open club
Contact:rolandsoong@centralparktc.org

Front Runners
Gay and lesbian running club, Manhattan
Contact: (212) 724-9700
chtorr@interport.net

Greater Long Island Running Club
Open club based in Long Island
Contact: (516) 349-7646

Greater New York Racing Team
Premier city club; head coach is also the NYCM's official coach and best-selling author.
Contact: CoachBobGlover@aol.com

Millrose Athletic Association
Long-standing Manhattan-based open club
Contact: david@millroseaa.org

Moving Comfort New York
Competitive Manhattan women-only team
Contact: (212) 737-4702
candestickles@worldnet.att.net

New York Flyers
Named Manhattan's most social running team
Contact: mal@nyflyers.org

New York Harriers
Calls itself a drinking club with a running problem
Contact: Douglas Hegley at nyharriers@yahoo.com

Prospect Park Track Club
Based in Prospect Park, Brooklyn
Contact: (718) 595-2049
www.pptc.org

Quantum Feet Road Runners Club
Based in Queens

Contact: (718) 454-3338
qtmfeet@aol.com

Staten Island Athletic Club
Based in Clove Lakes Park, Staten Island
Contact: Andy Burek at Siac7@aol.com

Taconic Road Runners Club
Based in Yorktown
Contact: Greg Diamond at greg@runner.org

Urban Athletics Running Team
Manhattan-based store/club, "Best deals and running advice for any tourist"
Contact: Jerry Macari at (212) 570-6069

Van Cortlandt Track Club
Bronx-based open running club
Contact: Bill Gaston at gastonb@iimagazine.com

Warren Street Social & Athletic Club
Manhattan-based competitive club
Contact: Rick Pascarella at rickpascarella@msn.com

West Side Runners
Manhattan-based open club
Contact: Bill Staab at (212) 787-4775

New York Running Stores

Gubbins Running Ahead
86 Park Place
East Hampton, NY 11937
(631) 329-7678
and
7 Windmill Lane
Southampton, NY 11968
(631) 287-4945

Jim Dalberth Sporting Goods
926 Genesee Street
Rochester, NY 14611
(716) 328-9746

M. Medved Co., Inc.
3400 Monroe Avenue
Rochester, NY 14618
(716) 248-3420
m.medved1@netscape.net

Paragon Athletic
Paragon provides free buses from the expo to the store during Marathon
Week.
867 Broadway
New York, NY 10003
(212) 255-8036
www.paragonsports.com

Quantum Feet
188-13 Union Turnpike
Fresh Meadows, NY 11366
(718) 454-3338
www.quantumfeet.com
qtmfet@aol.com
and
7 Windmill Lane
Southampton, NY 11968
(631) 287-4945

Runner's Edge
294 Main St.
Farmingdale, NY 11735
(516) 420-7963
www.runnersedge.com

Runner's Roost
4190 N. Buffalo Blvd.

Orchard Park, NY 14127
(716) 662-1331
and
410 Abbott Road
Buffalo, NY 14220
(716) 821-0008
www.teamroost.com

The Running Start
2113 Ave. U
Brooklyn, NY 11229
(718) 934-9113

The Sporting Foot
3401 Erie Blvd.
Ames Plaza
Dewitt, NY 13214
(315) 446-7342

Super Runners Shop
Former NYC Marathon Champion Gary Muhrcke owns a number of stores
in Manhattan and one on Long Island.

Manhattan
Grand Central Terminal, (646) 487-1120
360 Amsterdam Ave. (at 77th St.), (212) 787-7665
1337 Lexington Ave. (at 89th St.), (212) 369-6010
1246 Third Ave. (at 72nd St.), (212) 249-2133

Long Island
355 New York Ave., Huntington, NY 11743, (631) 549-3006
www.superrunnersshop.com

Westchester Road Runner
179 E. Post Road
White Plains, NY 10601
(914) 682-0637
www.wrrunner@aol.com

Sports Doctors and Other Experts

HAROLD ACHILLE, L.M.T.
Licensed Sports Massage Therapist
(718) 657-6206
(718) 600-6235
 Works at more than forty races per year helping athletes with pre/post-race massages. Elite Athlete Masseur for the New York City Marathon.

TZVI BARAK, P.T., Ph.D., O.C.S.
Physical Therapist
1015 Madison Avenue
New York, NY 10021
(212) 772-6610
 Specializing in treatment and prevention of running injuries.

LOUIS T. CALVANO
Chiropractor
4 East 89th Street
New York, NY 10128
(212) 369-5490
 A former sub-2:20 marathoner with more than fourteen years of experience.

JOHN CONNORS, DPM, FACFO
Podiatric Medicine and Surgery, Sports Medicine
Lexington Professional Center
133 East 73rd Street
New York, NY 10021
(212) 861-9000
 The choice of all the top Kenyan athletes coming to the New York City Marathon.
 "John is very able—he sorts out all my running problems."—Tegla Loroupe, two-time winner of the New York City Marathon.
 "Usually during marathon week I can fit anyone in at a moment's notice if they need help," says John.

LAURA A. FAVIN, L.M.T.
New York–Licensed Massage Therapist
324 West 89th Street #3A
New York, NY 10024
(212) 501-0606
  Swedish, Deep Tissue, Triggerpoint Therapy, and Medical Massage.

GARY J. FLORIO, M.D.
Sports and Entertainment Physicians, P.C.
244 West 54th Street
New York, NY 10019
(212) 262-9178
  The office is above Gold's Gym, with other therapists working on board.

GARY P. GUERRIERO, P.T., P.C.
515 Madison Avenue
(212) 355-8440
  The U.S. Athletic Training Center's head physical therapist.
  One of the city's best; works with a host of elite athletes.

RICHARD A. IZZO, D.C., C.C.S.P.
Chiropractor
10 Rye Ridge Plaza
Suite 210
Rye Brook, NY 10573
(914) 251-1223
  New York City Marathon finisher, 1988–92.

DANIEL HAMNER, M.D.
M.D. physiatrist, accupuncturist
  "Minimum of one hour" hands-on approach by one of the city's top
masters runners.
3 E. 71st Street
New York, NY 10021
(212) Pep-1991

LEWIS G. MAHARAM, M.D., FACSM
Medical Director of the New York City Marathon
24 W. 57th Street
New York, NY 10019
(212) 308-2348

BRUCE MANDELBAUM, L.Ac.
Sports acupunturist, massage therapist
2121 Broadway, Suite 401A
New York, NY 10023
(212) 769-4295
    A longtime member of the NYC running scene, with more than twenty
years of hands-on experience.

ANA J. SANZ, DPM
    Works alongside John Connors (see above).

AMANDA SCOLA, L.M.T.
Sports Massage
15 West 72nd Street
New York, NY 10023
(212) 724-5476
    Active Isolated Stretching techniques. Certified in Neuromuscular
Therapy and Pregnancy Massage.

Jim and Phil Wharton
Active Isolated Flexibility
After Khalid Khannouchi set the men's world record in the spring of 2002, he
thanked the Whartons for helping him achieve the result.
51 W. 81st Street
New York, NY 10024
(212) 799-7559

Running-Related Web Links

RACES AND RACING

www.nyrrc.org
The New York Road Runners Club

www.nycmarathon.org
The New York City Marathon's official site

baa.org
The Boston Marathon's official site

www.chicagomarathon.com
The site for the Chicago Marathon

www.londomarathon.co.uk
The official site of the London Marathon

www.runningtimes.com
American running magazine

www.marathonguide.com
A site for marathon runners

www.runnersworld.com
Web site of the world's most popular running magazine

www.raceresultsweekly.com
Running results from races worldwide

www.coolrunning.com
Web magazine for runners

www.agemasters.com
Gives age-equivalent performances for sporting feats

EQUIPMENT AND APPAREL

www.nike.com
Sporting giant

www.asics.com
Japanese sporting company

www.mizuno.com
Japanese sporting company

www.newbalance.com
American running shoe and clothing company

www.saucony.com
American running shoe and clothing company

www.roadrunnersports.com
Web running store

www.adidas.com
Another sporting giant

MORE USEFUL NYC WEB LINKS

Metropolitan Transit Authority (MTA)
Train, subway, and bus maps and schedules for all of Manhattan and the
surrounding boroughs.
www.mta.nyc.ny.us/

Most New York
Web Site of the *New York Daily News*. First-rate source for news, sports,
gossip, entertainment, and film and restaurant reviews.
www.mostnewyork.com/

NY Bytes
Food and restaurants forum covering restaurants and caterers in
New York City.
www.nybytes.com/

TravelPackets.com
Sign up to receive a free packet of information, including maps, brochures,
and discount coupons—everything you need for planning a trip to NYC.
new-york.travelpackets.com

NYC hotel and travel services
www.hoteldiscounts.com

NYC shopping sites
www.theinsider.com/nyc/links/link4.htm

NYC travel information
www.budgettravel.com/

Central Web site for NYC
www.ny.com/

General information about the city
newyork.citysearch.com

Plug in a zip code and get a location
www.ny.com/locator/

A guide to the city's sights and attractions
www.ny.com/sights/misc.html

NYC Tourist Phone Numbers

Avery Fisher Hall	Lincoln Center	(212) 875-5030
Carnegie Hall	57th Street and 7th Avenue	(212) 247-7800
Metropolitan Opera	Lincoln Center	(212) 362-6000
NY Visitors Bureau	2 Columbus Circle	(212) 397-8222
Radio City Music Hall	50th Street and 6th Avenue	(212) 247-4777

Shea Stadium	126th Street and Roosevelt Avenue	(718) 507-8499
Yankee Stadium	161st & River Ave.	(718) 293-6000

Airports

JFK	(718) 244-4444
La Guardia	(718) 533-3400
Newark	(201) 961-2000

NYC Transportation Phone Numbers

Subway and Bus info	(718) 330-1234
Amtrak	(800) 872-7245
Greyhound	(212) 971-6363
Metro North	(212) 532-4900
New Jersey Transit	(201) 762-5100
New York City Port Authority	(212) 564-8484
Staten Island Ferry	(212) 806-6940
Staten Island Rapid Transit	(718) 447-8601
Statue of Liberty Ferry	(718) 390-5253

Index

Page numbers in **bold** indicate tables.

A (anaerobic-threshold-pace), 35
ABC television airing of NYCM, 12
Abebe Bikila Award, 143
Achille, Harold, 26
Aesop's Tables, 93
Africans in NYCM, 13, 15–16
Afternoon for buying running shoes, 3
Age requirements for NYCM, 24
Airports, 52, 178
Aleve, 136
Alexis, Kim, 163
Allen, Woody, 55
Alley Pond Park, 76
Amateur Athletic Union, 9
American food in NYC, 92
Americans in NYCM, 9, 10, 11, 12
Anaerobic-threshold-pace (A), 35
Anti-inflammatory pills, 136
Apartments, furnished, 61
Appearance money, 19–20
Aquino, Claudia, 157
Armstrong, Natalie, 157
Arturo's, 87
Attractions of New York City, 143–59
Au Bon Pain, 83
Australians in NYCM, 14

Authorized tour operators, 24
"Ax" (ask) (NYC speak), 89

Baci Italian, 91
Bagelry, The, 86
Bagels, 83–86
Bagels on the Square, 83
Baggage-truck crew (volunteers), 28
Balanced diet, 41, 42–44, 45, 46, 105
Base-work running, 34
Bayo, Zebedayo, 17, 33
Bay Ridge Bike and Pedestrian Path, 71
Beauty products, avoiding, 106
Bed for recovery, 136
Beginners' Running Program, 5. *See also*
    Running, beginning
Belvedere, 56
Benefits of running, 1
Bentley, Philip, 157
Bethpage Bike Path, 78–79
Bialy (NYC speak), 89
Blackford, Andy, 122
Blondies, 139
Bloomberg, Mike, 55
Blue group of NYCM, 101, 104
Blue number family reunion area, 124

Bonner, Beth, 9, 161
Bordin, Gelindo, 47
Boroughs of NYC
    NYCM and, 10–11
    spectating by, 113–17, **115–17**
    See also Running in NYC; Travel
        accommodations
Boulevard Motor Inn, Queens, 60
Boyer, Blair, 141
Brantly, Keith, 15
Brazilian food in NYC, 95
Breakfast nutrition, 98, 103, 106
Breal, Michael, xiv
Breathing of skin, 106, 119, 134
Bridle Path (Central Park), 66
British in NYCM, 12, 13, 14
Bronx, The
    food in, 93
    NYCM (course), 122
    running in, 77–78
    spectating in, 114
Bronx Half-Marathon, 164
Bronx Zoo, 144
Brooklyn
    food in, 94
    NYCM (course), 121
    running in, 70–73
    spectating in, 114
Brooklyn Bridge, 72
Brooklyn Half-Marathon, 163
Brooklyn Heights Promenade, 73
Burfoot, Amby, 33
Bus loaders (volunteers), 28
Busses for travel, 52, 97

Cadman Plaza, 73
Café Fiorello, 91
Café Lalo, 139
Café Mozart, 138–39
Cafeteria, 90
Campbell, John, 162
Canceling entry in NYCM, 25
Carbohydrate loading, 46, 47, 105
Carbohydrates, 41, 43, 45
Cardiovascular system and training, 33
Carey Wall Street 4.01 Rat Race, 163
Carlisle, Kitty, 55
Cars to get to starting line, 97–98

Cathedral St. John the Divine, 144–45
Catuna, Anuta, 16, 165
Central Park
    description of, 54, 145–46
    NYCM and, xv, 9–10
    running in, 64–67
Central Park Wildlife Center and Zoo, 146
Ceron, Dionicio, 44
Challenges of training, 33–34
ChampionChip, 17, 28, 102–3, 123
Cheaper alternatives to travel, 60–61
Chebet, Joseph, 17, 39, 165
Chelsea, 53, 56–57
Chepchumba, Joyce, 19, 25–27, 105, 137
Chepkemei, Susan, 26, 27
Cheslik, Tom, xv
Chinatown, 53
Chinese food in NYC, 94
Chrysler Building, 147
City Hall Park, 146–47
Clarion, 57
Clothing for running
    beginning running and, 3
    layering clothing, 3, 100
    pre-checking and race day, 98
    starting line, 98, 99–101, 106
    temperature, 3, 100–101, 106, 128–29
Clothing for spectators, 111–12
Clove Lakes Park, 74–75
Coffee, 87
Columbus Bakery, 139
Commitment to training, 38–41
Condor, Ernest, 111
Conley, John, 156
Consistency for running, 6
Cook, Robin, 56
Cooking with Jazz, 93–94
Cooldown, 4, 35
CoolMax, 3, 100
Corner Bistro, 90
Course of NYCM, 121–28
Course records of NYCM, 11, 12, 13, 14, 22, 117, 161–62
Courtney, Dave, 158
Crocodile Dundee, 55
Cronkite, Walter, 55
"Cross-trainers" shoes, 2
Cross-training (XT), 35

Da Silvano, 91
Davis, Sammy Jr., 55
Days Hotel, 60
Debuts in NYCM, fastest, 11–12, 14
Deferral service, 25
Dehydration, 33, 34, 131. *See also* Water
    drinking
Denino's Pizzeria/Tavern, 88
Department of Consumer Affairs, 62
Desire to run, 32
Diamond, Neil, 55
Dieker, Anke, 157
Diner, 91
Dining
    NYCM, dining after, 138–40
    restaurant tips, 81–82
    See also Food in NYC
Disabled athletes, 22, 105
Distance, building up, 33
Districts of Manhattan, 52–55
Dixon, Rod, 12
Downtown Manhattan, 52–53
Drossin, Deena, 27
Dyker Beach Golf Course, 71–72

Early starts to NYCM, 105
East (even-numbered streets), 52
East Side, 51
East Village, 53
Easy running (Es), 35
Eating. *See* Dining; Food in NYC; Nutrition
Economic impact of NYCM, 19
Edgar's Café, 139
Elite men/women in NYCM, 104, 105, 134
Ellis Island and Statue of Liberty, 147
El Mouaziz, Abdelkhader, 18
Empire, 57–58
Empire State Building, 147–48
Energy waves, 34
Entering the NYCM, 21–30
    age requirements for, 24
    authorized tour operators and, 24
    baggage-truck crew, 28
    bus loaders, 28
    canceling entry, 25
    deferral service, 25
    Exposition, 29–30
    family reunion helpers, 28
    finish-line workers, 28

fourth-try guaranteed entry, 24
guaranteed entries, 24, 25
half-marathon qualifying times, 23
hand-crank division, 22, 105
lottery for, 21–22, 24
New York City Marathon Exposition,
    29–30
NYRR race participation for, 23
photo identification for, 29, 30
qualifying times for, 23
race packages, distribution of, 29
race veterans and, 24
registration acceptance card, 29, 30
tour operators (authorized) and, 24
veterans of NYCM, 24
volunteering, 28–29
water station workers, 28
wheelchair division, 22, 105
Entrants (number of) NYCM, 9, 10, 13
Erikson, Åke, 33
Es (easy running), 35
Espinosa, Andres, 15, 44
ESPN Zone, 140
Ess-A-Bagel, 83–84
Essex House, 58
Ethiopians in NYCM, 19
Ethnic cuisines, 94–95
Evans, Paul, 32
EWR (Newark Int.), 52
Exposition, 29–30

F (Fartlek) (speed-play), 35
Facts and figures of NYCM, 9–19, 161–65
Facts on New York City, 52
Family Reunion Area, 124
Family reunion helpers (volunteers), 28
Fartlek (speed-play) (F), 35
Fat, 41, 43, 45
Father of the Modern Marathon (Fred
    Lebow), 7, 10–11, 14, 15, 16, 55, 64, 119
Favorite foods, 44–45
Favorite things to do in NYC, 156–58
Fernandez, Adriana, 18
Fiacconi, Franca, 17, 165
Fiber, 43
Financial District, 52
Finishing Stretch of NYCM, 123
Finish Line of NYCM, 123–24
Finish-line workers (volunteers), 28

Finish of NYCM, closest, 17
Fiorello La Guardia Int. (LGA), 52
First race, 6
Fitzpatrick Grand Central, 58–59
Five-Mile Lower Loop (Central Park), 65
Five-Mile Upper Loop (Central Park), 65
Fleming, Tom, 9, 10, 63, 161, 162
Fluid stations in NYCM, 131–34
Flushing Meadows Park, 76
Flying kilometers, 32
Fonseca, Peter, xiii
Food in NYC, 81–95
    American, 92
    bagels, 83–86
    Brazilian, 95
    Bronx, The, 93
    Brooklyn, 94
    Chinese, 94
    coffee, 87
    dining after NYCM, 138–40
    dining tips, 81–82
    ethnic cuisines, 94–95
    French, 94
    hamburgers, 90–91
    Indian, 94
    Italian, 91–92, 94
    pizza, 87–89
    prices, 81
    Queens, 93–94
    reservations, 82
    "rush," 82
    seating waits, 82
    smoke-free zone, 82
    South American/Mexican, 95
    speaking New York, 89
    special needs and, 82
    Staten Island, 93
    tips, 82
    See also Nutrition
Forest Park, 75–76
Form for running (natural), 4
Foster, Brendan, 7
Four-hour schedule, training, 34, **36–37**
Four-Mile Loop (Central Park), 65
Fourth-try guaranteed entry, 24
Fred Lebow Classic 5–Miler, 163
French food in NYC, 94

Fridgeirsson, Stefan, 135
Fun and training, 32
"Fun Pass" MetroCard, 112

Garcia, Jose, 156
García, Salvador, 14
Garfunkel, Art, 122
Gatorade, 132
Germans in NYCM, 15
Get-U-Round (GUR) schedule, training, 34, 35, **36–37**
Giuliani, Rudy, 147
Glycogen levels and training, 34
Goal marathon-pace runs (MP), 35
Gomez, Rodolfo, 18, 165
Gorman, Miki, 11, 161
Gracie Mansion, 148
Gramercy Bagels, 84
Gramercy Park, 53
Grand Central Terminal, 148
Grant, Carey, 60
Grant's Tomb, 148–49
Great Lawn (Central Park), 66
Green group of NYCM, 101, 104, 105
Green number family reunion area, 124
Green Tree, The, 86
Greenwich Village
    description of, 51, 53
    running in, 70
Grimaldi's, 88
Guaranteed entries, 24, 25
GUR (Get-U-Round) schedule, training, 34, 35, **36–37**

H (hills), 35
Habitat Hotel, 60
Half-marathon qualifying times, 23
Hamburgers, 90–91
Hand-crank division, NYCM, 22, 105
Hannah, Darryl, 162
Hard Rock Café, 92
Harlem
    description of, 55
    NYCM (course), 122–23
    running in, 70
Harlem Y, 61
Hayes, Tom, 68
Healthy Bagel, 84
Heel of running shoes, 3

Hellebuyck, Eddy, 32, 44, 134
Hemingway, Mariel, 163
Higgins, Norman, 161
Hill, Ron, 39
Hills (H), 35
Hilton Hotel, 25, 27
History of NYCM, 9–20
Holiday Inn, Midtown, 61
Holiday Inn, SoHo, 61
Home Alone, 55
Horne, Lena, 55
Hot and Crusty Bagels, 84
Hot Bagels, 84
Hot Chocolate 15K, 164
Hotels, 56–61
Hotel slouch's spectating, 107, 108
Hughes, Langston, 55
Hussein, Ibrahim, 13, 16
Hydration, 131–34. *See also* Water drinking

Ibuprofen, 136
"I can" person from running, 1
Ice for sore parts, 136, 137
Ikangaa, Juma, 14, 32–33, 39, 42, 162
Inaugural New York City Marathon, 9
Indian food in NYC, 94
Information Center, 51
Injuries from running, 6, 7
InterContinental, 59
International Amateur Athletic Federation, 43
International Friendship Run, 21, 143
Internationality of NYCM, 11, 12, 13
Interval training at VO$_2$ (V), 35
Inwood, 55
Island Burgers & Shakes, 90
Italian food in NYC, 91–92, 94
Italians in NYCM, 13, 16, 17

Jackson Hole, 90
Jacob K. Javits Center (Marketplace for the World), 29, 149
"Jeet?" (NYC speak), 89
JFK (John F. Kennedy Int.), 52
Jifar, Tesfaye, 19, 117–18, 162
Joe Allen, 90
Joel, Billy, 55
Joe's Pizza, 88
Johanssen, Ingemar, 163

John F. Kennedy Int. (JFK), 52
Johnson, Lars-Åke, 157
John's Pizza, 88
Jones, Hugh, 12, 41, 136–37
Jones, Kim, 40, 164
Jones, Steve, 13
Junior's, 92

Kagwe, John, xiv, 16–17, 158–59, 165
Kenyans in NYCM, 13, 15–16, 16–17, 17–18, 19
Kessler, Ben "Pizza," 88
Khannouchi, Khalid, 79
Killy, Jean-Claude, 163
Kimani, Joseph, 31
Kipkoech, Paul, 32
Kiplagat, Esther, 26
Kiplagat, Lornah, 44
Kissena Park, 76
Knish (NYC speak), 89
Krebs, Peter, 72
Kristiansen, Ingrid, 14
Kurtis, Doug, 32

Lactic acid, 135
Lagat, Elijah, 40
La Guardia, Fiorello H., 148
Langat, Steven, 32
Langerhorst, Pieter, 129
La Pizza Fresca Ristorante, 88–89
Last few days diet, 48, 105–6
Last-minute reminders, 105–6
Late Night with Conan O'Brian, 156
Late Show with David Letterman, 156
Lauren, Ralph, 162
Lawson, Jerry, 33, 39
Layering clothing, 3, 100
Lebow, Fred (Father of the Modern Marathon), 7, 10–11, 14, 15, 16, 55, 64, 119
Lee, General Robert E., 121
Leghzaoui, Asmae, 163
Lennon, John, 154
Lenny's Bagels, 85
Lenox, 138
Leone, Giacomo, 16
Leppin Sports, 44
LGA (Fiorello La Guardia Int.), 52
Lincoln Center of Performing Arts, 149

Little Italy, 53
Lobster Box, 93
London Marathon, 12
Long distance, avoiding obsession, 32
Long Island running, 78–79
Loroupe, Tegla, 15–16, 25, 41, 47, 126
Lottery for entering NYCM, 21–22, 24
Lower East Side, 53
Lower East Side Pedestrian Pathways, 67–68

Madison Avenue Bridge, 113, 122
Madison Hotel, 61
Madonna, 56, 57, 162
Magnusdottir, Bryndis, 157
Maher, Peter, 128
Main race of NYCM, 104
Malinin, Mike, 162
Maloney, Michael, 157
Mama Leone's, 124
Manhattan
    NYCM (course), 122
    returning to (spectators), 114–15
    running in, 63–70
    spectating in, 114
    See also Travel accommodations
Manhattan Half-Marathon, 164
Man-made fibers, 3, 100
Mantle, Mickey, 55–56
Marathon, xiv. *See also* New York City
    Marathon (NYCM)
Marathon Celebration Party, 136, 138
Marco Polo, 94
Marcos, Imelda, 55
Marketplace for the World (Jacob K. Javits
    Center), 29, 149
Massage for recovery, 136–37
Mayflower, 59–60
McCarren Park, 72
McCartney, Paul, 162
McColgan, Liz, 14
McKiernan, Catherina, 32, 45
McPherson, Elle, 55
Meltzer, Gary, 24
Mercedes-Benz, 13, 15
Merritt, Kim, 10, 161
Metropolitan Museum of Art, 149–50
Mexicans in NYCM, 14, 15, 18
Midtown East Side, 54
Midtown Manhattan, 54

Midtown West Side, 54
Mile, calories burned running per, 45
Mileage, increasing, 6
Minerals, 43
Monti, David, 19–20
Moore, Mary Tyler, 55
MP (goal marathon-pace runs), 35
Mtolo, Willie, 14
Muhrcke, Gary, 9, 47, 161
Multiple marathons, 137–38
Multi-spot plan spectating, 109–12
Murray's Bagels, 85
Museum of Modern Art, 150
Mustang Sally's Saloon, 140
Mykytok, Mike, 157
Mylar blankets, 11, 28, 123, 129

NASDAQ MarketSite, 150
National anthem, 104
Natural-based diets, 43–44
Natural form for running, 4
Ndereba, Catherine, 18
Newark Int. (EWR), 52
New York Aquarium, 150–51
New York Botanical Gardens, 78, 151
New York City Marathon Exposition, 29–30
New York City Marathon (NYCM), 9–20
    ABC television airing of, 12
    Allan Steinfeld, 16, 18, 19–20, 99
    appearance money, 19–20
    boroughs of New York and, 10–11
    Central Park and, xv, 9–10
    ChampionChip, 17, 28, 102–3, 123
    course records, 11, 12, 13, 14, 22, 117,
        161–62
    debuts, fastest-ever, 11–12, 14
    economic impact of, 19
    entrants (number of), 9, 10, 13
    facts and figures, 9–19, 161–65
    finish, closest, 17
    Fred Lebow (Father of the Modern
        Marathon) and, 7, 10–11, 14, 15, 16, 55,
        64, 119
    history of, 9–20
    inaugural NYCM, 9
    internationality of, 11, 12, 13
    Mylar blankets, 11, 28, 123, 129
    non-American winner, first, 12
    performance-related prize money, 11

planning for, 19–20
professionalism of, 9, 11
race directors, 7, 10–11, 14, 15, 16, 18, 19–20
short-course records, 12, 13
sponsor of, 13, 15
sub-2:20 marathons, 10, 32
terrorist attacks (9/11), 18–19
three-hour barrier and women, 9, 10
three wins in a row, 11, 12
toilets, 41, 98–99, 103
weather and, 10, 14, 15, 19, 128–29
Web site for, 21
winning margins (closest), 164–65
women's race, starting of, 9
"Wrong-Way Silva," 15, 165
See also Entering the NYCM; Food in NYC; Race, the; Recovery; Running, beginning; Running in NYC; Spectators; Starting line, getting to; Training for the marathon; Travel accommodations
New York City (NYC)
attractions, 143–59
economic impact of NYCM, 19
facts on, 52
favorite things to do in, 156–58
races in, 163–64
resources, 167–78
running stores, 169–71
speaking NYC, 89
survival tips for, 62–63
tourist phone numbers, 177–78
transportation phone numbers, 178
See also Food in NYC; New York City Marathon (NYCM); Running in NYC; Travel accommodations
New York Public Library, 151
New York's Mini Marathon, 163
New York Times, 153
New Zealanders in NYCM, 12
No Idea, 140
Non-American winner (first) in NYCM, 12
Non-running days, 32
Norwegians in NYCM, 11, 12, 13, 14
Novotel, 61
Nutrition, 41–49
balanced diet, 41, 42–44, 45, 46, 105
carbohydrate loading, 46, 47, 105

carbohydrates, 41, 43, 45
fat, 41, 43, 45
favorite foods, 44–45
fiber, 43
last few days diet, 48, 105–6
mile, calories burned per, 45
minerals, 43
natural-based diets, 43–44
Pasta Party at Tavern on the Green, 49
protein, 41, 43, 45
recovery and, 46, 135–36, 137, 138–40
spicy food, avoiding, 32
"squeezy," 44
supplements, 42, 44, 46
sweating and water drinking, 42
urine color and water drinking, 42
vegetarians, 46
water drinking, 33, 34, 41–42, 43, 46
women and, 46
See also Food in NYC; Training for the marathon
NYC. *See* New York City
NYCM. *See* New York City Marathon
NYRR, 22, 23, 29, 66, 133, 163, 164

Okayo, Margaret, 18, 19, 20, 161
Olmstead, Frederick Law, 70, 145
Olsen, Rolf, 158
Olympic Games of 1896, xiv
Onassis, Jackie, 55
Ondieki, Lisa, 14, 74, 161
One-spot guide to spectating, 107, 108
Orientation in Manhattan, 51–52
Orthotics, 4
O'Shea, Shirley, 158

Pace
consistency for NYCM, 119
training, 32–33, 38, **38**
Pacino, Al, 55
Panfil, Wanda, 14, 164
Paredes, Benjamin, 15, 165
Park Avalon, 92
Partner for running, 4, 34, 98
Pasta d'Oro, 26, 27
Pasta Party at Tavern on the Green, 49
Patience for running, 4, 33
Payard's Pâtisserie, 138
Performance-related prize money, 11

Pero, Anthony "Totonno," 89
Petrova, Ludmila, 18, 136, 165
Pheidippides, xiv
Photo identification for NYCM, 29, 30
Pick-A-Bagel, 85
Pink number family reunion area, 124
Pippig, Uta, 15
Pizza, 87–89
Pizzolato, Orlando, 13
Planning for NYCM, 19–20
Plan (training), following, 33
Poitier, Sidney, 55
Poli, Gianni, 13
Polish in NYCM, 14
Pomodoro Rosso, 91–92
Porta Potties, 98–99, 103
Pre-race tips for NYCM, 120
Prices of food in NYC, 81
Professionalism of NYCM, 9, 11
Prospect Park Wildlife Center, 151–52
Protein, 41, 43, 45
Pulaski Bridge, 113, 121, 125, 130

Qualifying times for NYCM, 23
Queens
    food in, 93–94
    NYCM (course), 121–22
    running in, 75–76
    spectating in, 114
Queensborough Bridge, 113, 122, 126, 130
Queens Half-Marathon, 163
Queens Wildlife Center, 152
Quinn, Anthony, 55

R (Race), 35
Race, first, 6
Race, The, 119–34
    Bronx, The (course), 122
    Brooklyn (course), 121
    course, 121–28
    elite men and women, 104, 105, 134
    Family Reunion Area, 124
    Finishing Stretch, 123
    Finish Line, 123–24
    fluid stations, 131–34
    Harlem (course), 122–23
    hydration, 131–34
    Manhattan (course), 122
    Mylar blankets, 11, 28, 123, 129
    pace consistency for, 119
    pre-race tips, 120
    Queensborough Bridge (course), 122
    Queens (course), 121–22
    Return to Manhattan (course), 122–23
    skin breathing, 106, 119, 134
    Sponge Station, 119, 134
    starting line, getting to, 98–99
    Staten Island (start), 121
    Sweep Bus, 128
    temperature, 3, 100–101, 106, 128–29
    training tips, 40
    undulation profile of, 129–30
    "Wall," hitting the, 122, 126
    water drinking plan, 119, 131–34
    weather and, 10, 14, 15, 19, 128–29
    See also New York City Marathon (NYCM)
Race busses to get to starting line, 97
Race directors of NYCM, 7, 10–11, 14, 15, 16, 18, 19–20
Race pace and training, 32–33
Race packages, distribution of, 29
Race (R), 35
Races in NYC, 163–64. *See also* New York City Marathon (NYCM)
Race veterans and NYCM, 24
Rasputin, 94
Recovery, 135–42
    anti-inflammatory pills, 136
    bed, 136
    dining after the marathon, 138–40
    ice for sore parts, 136, 137
    lactic acid, 135
    Marathon Celebration Party, 136, 138
    massage, 136–37
    multiple marathons, 137–38
    nutrition, 46, 135–36, 137, 138–40
    Runner's Rigor Mortis, 135
    sleep, 137
    sore parts, 136, 137
    Sports Bars (Manhattan), 139–40
    stretching, 4, 137
    Upper East Side dining, 138
    Upper West Side dining, 138–40
    walking, 135, 136, 137
    water drinking, 136
    water therapy, 136, 137
Red group of NYCM, 101, 104
Red Hook Track, 73

Red number family reunion area, 124
Registration acceptance card, 29, 30
Religious services, 104
Reservations for dining, 82
Reservoir (Central Park), 65–66
Restaurant Guides, 82
Return policies for running shoes, 4
Return to Manhattan (course), 122–23
Rewarding yourself, 4
Riverdale Park, 78
Rivers, Joan, 55
Riverside Church, 152
Roberto's, 93
Roberts, Robin, 78
Rochat-Moser, Franziska, 17
Rockefeller Estate, 79
Rockfeller Center, 152
Rodgers, Bill, 11, 100, 132, 162
Roe, Allison, 12, 161
Ronald McDonald House Kids' Half-Mile
    Fun Run, 144
Roosevelt Island Tramway, 152–53
Rop, Rodgers, 27
Rossellini, Isabella, 55
Rossettie, Michelle, 85
Roth, David Lee, 163
Rumanians in NYCM, 16
Runner's Rigor Mortis, 135
Runners' timetable, **115–17**
Runner's World, 122
Running, beginning, 1–7
    afternoon for buying running shoes, 3
    Beginners' Running Program, 5
    beginner tips, 4
    benefits of, 1
    clothing for, 3
    consistency for, 6
    cooldown, 4, 35
    first race, 6
    form for running (natural), 4
    heel of running shoes, 3
    "I can" person from, 1
    injuries, 6, 7
    layering clothing, 3, 100
    man-made fibers, 3
    mileage, increasing, 6
    orthotics, 4
    patience for, 4, 33
    race, first, 6

return policies for running shoes, 4
rewarding yourself, 4
"running niggle," 7
running shoes, 2–3
steps per mile, 155
stretching, 4, 137
support for, 4, 34, 98
temperature and running clothing, 3
toe room in running shoes, 3
walking, alternating with, 4
warmup, 4, 35
See also Training for the marathon
Running in NYC, 63–79
    Alley Pond Park, 76
    Bay Ridge Bike and Pedestrian Path, 71
    Bethpage Bike Path, 78–79
    Bridle Path (Central Park), 66
    Bronx, The, 77–78
    Brooklyn, 70–73
    Brooklyn Bridge, 72
    Brooklyn Heights Promenade, 73
    Cadman Plaza, 73
    Central Park, 64–67
    Clove Lakes Park, 74–75
    clubs, 167–69
    Dyker Beach Golf Course, 71–72
    Five-Mile Lower Loop (Central Park), 65
    Five-Mile Upper Loop (Central Park), 65
    Flushing Meadows Park, 76
    Forest Park, 75–76
    Four-Mile Loop (Central Park), 65
    Great Lawn (Central Park), 66
    Greenwich Village, 70
    Harlem, 70
    Kissena Park, 76
    Long Island, 78–79
    Lower East Side Pedestrian Pathways,
        67–68
    Manhattan, 63–70
    McCarren Park, 72
    New York Botanical Gardens, 78, 151
    Queens, 75–76
    Red Hook Track, 73
    Reservoir (Central Park), 65–66
    Riverdale Park, 78
    Rockefeller Estate, 79
    Six-Mile Loop (Central Park), 65
    SoHo, 70
    Staten Island, 73–75

Running in NYC (*cont.*)
    Triangle below Canal (TriBeCa), 70
    Upper East Side, 69–70
    Upper West Side, 68–69
    Van Cortlandt Park Run, 77, 164
    Westchester County, 79
    West Side, 63–64
    See also Travel accommodations
"Running niggle," 7
Running-related Web sites, 175–76
Running shoes
    afternoon for buying, 3
    beginning running and, 2–3
    heel of, 3
    return policies for, 4
    starting line and, 106
    toe room in, 3
    training and, 33
Running stores (NYC), 169–71
Runyan, Marla, 105
"Rush" times (dining), 82
Russ and Daughters, 85
Russians in NYCM, 18
Rye Playland, 153

Saint Patrick's Cathedral, 153
Salazar, Alberto, 11, 12, 124, 162, 165
Samuelson, Joan Benoit, 118
Sanders, Summer, 162
Sang, Patrick, 17
Saturday Night Live, 156
Schedules for training, 35–37, **36–37**
Schmear (NYC speak), 89
Seating waits (dining), 82
Serendipity, 139
Sex in the City, 125
Shahanga, Gidamis, 39
Shoes. *See* Running shoes
Short-course records of NYCM, 12, 13
Shorter, Frank, 134
Shorts, 99, 100
Silva, German, 15, 16, 17, 165
Simon, Paul, 122
Sinatra, Frank, 55
Singlets, 99, 100
Six-Mile Loop (Central Park), 65
Skin breathing, 106, 119, 134
Slater, Christian, 162
Sleep for recovery, 137

Sleepless in Seattle, 147
Smith, Geoff, 12
Smoke-free zone of restaurants, 82
Snowflake 4–Miler, 163
SoHo, 53, 70
Sore parts, 136, 137
South Africans in NYCM, 14
South American/Mexican food in NYC, 95
South Street Seaport, 153–54
Speaking New York, 89
Special needs and dining in NYC, 82
Spectators, 107–18
    boroughs of NYC and, 113–17, **115–17**
    Bronx spectating, 114
    Brooklyn spectating, 114
    clothing, 111–12
    essentials for, 108, 112
    hotel slouch's guide, 107, 108
    Manhattan, returning to, 114–15
    Manhattan spectating, 114
    multi-spot plan, 109–12
    one-spot guide, 107, 108
    Queens spectating, 114
    runners' timetable, **115–17**
    spotting your runner, 112–13
    Staten Island spectating, 113–14
    subway travel for, 107–8, 109–12
    supplies for runners, 112, 130
    television, 107, 108
    two-spot guide, 109
Speed play (Fartlek, F), 35
Spence, Steve, 133
Spicy food, avoiding, 32
Sponge Station, 119, 134
Sponsor of NYCM, 13, 15
Sports Bars (Manhattan), 139–40
Sports doctors and experts, 172–74
Spotting your runner, 112–13
"Squeezy," 44
Starbucks, 87
Starting line, getting to, 97–106
    beauty products, avoiding, 106
    Blue group, 101, 104
    breakfast nutrition, 98, 103, 106
    busses, 97
    cars, 97–98
    ChampionChip, 17, 28, 102–3, 123
    clothing, 98, 99–101, 106
    clothing and baggage pre-checked, 98

disabled athletes, 105
early starts, 105
elite men and women, 104, 105, 134
Green group, 101, 104, 105
hand-crank division, 22, 105
last-minute reminders, 105–6
layering clothing, 3, 100
main race, 104
national anthem, 104
partner for, 98
race busses, 97
race day, 98–99
Red group, 101, 104
religious services, 104
running shoes, 106
starting areas, 101, 104
surviving the start, 103–5
taxis, 97–98
temperature, 3, 100–101, 106, 128–29
toilets, 41, 98–99, 103
UPS bags, 104
Vaseline for chafing, 104, 106
Verazzano-Narrows Bridge closing, 97
waking up, 98
warmup, 99–100, 106
wheelchair assistance, 97
wheelchair division, 22, 105
Staten Island
food in, 93
NYCM (start), 121
running in, 73–75
spectating in, 113–14
Staten Island Ferry, 154
Staten Island Half Marathon, 164
Staten Island Zoo, 154
Statue of Liberty, 147
Steinfeld, Allan, 16, 18, 19–20, 99
Steps per mile, 155
Stern, Howard, 162
Strawberry Fields, 154
Stretching, 4, 137
Sub-2:20 marathons, NYCM, 10, 32
Subway travel, 107–8, 109–12
Supplements, nutrition, 42, 44, 46
Supplies for runners, 112, 130
Support for running, 4, 34, 98
Survival tips for NYC, 62–63
Surviving the start of NYCM, 103–5
Sweating and water drinking, 42

Sweep Bus, 128
Swiss in NYCM, 17
Switzer, Katherine, 10
Szalkai, Anders, 157

Tal Bagels, 86
Tanui, Moses, 33, 39–40, 98, 134
Tanui, William, 46
Tanzanians in NYCM, 14
Tapering, 34
Tavern on the Green Pasta Party, 49
Taxis, 52, 97–98
Television shows in NYC, 156
Television spectating, 107, 108
Temperature and clothing, 3, 100–101, 106,
    128–29
Teodora, 92
Terrorist attacks (9/11), 18–19
Theater District, 155
Theodore Roosevelt House, 155
Three-hour barrier and women, 9, 10
Three-hour schedule, training, 34, **36–37**
Three wins in a row, NYCM, 11, 12
Time calculation for training, 31
Time Out, 140
Time predictor for training, 38, **38**
Times Square, 155
Timetable, runner, **115–17**
Tired legs, running on, 31
Today, 152, 156
Toe room in running shoes, 3
Toilets at NYCM, 41, 98–99, 103
Totonno's, 89
Tourist phone numbers (NYC), 177–78
Tour operators (authorized), 24
Training for the marathon, 31–49
    anaerobic-threshold-pace (A), 35
    base-work running, 34
    cardiovascular system, 33
    challenges, 33–34
    clothing for, 32
    commitment to, 38–41
    cooldown, 4, 35
    cross-training (XT), 35
    dehydration, 33, 34, 131
    desire to run, 32
    distance, building up, 33
    easy running (Es), 35
    energy waves, 34

Training for the marathon (*cont.*)
   Fartlek (speed-play) (F), 35
   flying kilometers, 32
   four-hour schedule, 34, **36–37**
   fun and, 32
   Get-U-Round (GUR) schedule, 34, 35,
     36–37
   glycogen levels, 34
   goal marathon-pace runs (MP), 35
   hills (H), 35
   interval training at VO_2 (V), 35
   long distance, avoiding obsession, 32
   non-running days, 32
   pace, 32–33, 38, **38**
   partner for, 34
   patience for, 4, 33
   plan, following, 33
   race day tips, 40
   race pace and, 32–33
   race (R), 35
   running shoes, 33
   schedules, 35–37, **36–37**
   tapering, 34
   three-hour schedule, 34, **36–37**
   time calculation for, 31
   time predictor, 38, **38**
   tired legs, running on, 31
   warmup, 4, 35
   water drinking, 33, 34, 41–42, 43, 46
   weather and, 33
   See also Nutrition; Running, beginning
Transportation phone numbers (NYC), 178
Trattoria Romana, 93
Trausti, Ivar, 44
Travel accommodations, 51–62
   airports, 52, 178
   apartments, furnished, 61
   busses, 52
   Central Park, 54
   cheaper alternatives, 60–61
   Chelsea, 53
   Chinatown, 53
   districts of Manhattan, 52–55
   Downtown Manhattan, 52–53
   east (even-numbered streets), 52
   East Side, 51
   East Village, 53
   Financial District, 52
   Gramercy Park, 53

Greenwich Village, 51, 53
Harlem, 55
hotels, 56–61
Information Center, 51
Inwood, 55
Little Italy, 53
Lower East Side, 53
Midtown East Side, 54
Midtown Manhattan, 54
Midtown West Side, 54
orientation in Manhattan, 51–52
SoHo, 53, 70
survival tips, 62–63
taxi services, 52
Triangle below Canal (TriBeCa), 53, 70
Upper East Side, 54, 55–56
Upper West Side, 54
Uptown Manhattan, 54
Washington Heights, 55
Washington Square, 51
Web sites for, 61
west (odd-numbered streets), 52
West Side, 51, 63–64
See also Running in NYC
Triangle below Canal (TriBeCa), 53, 70
Trinity Church, 155–56
Trujillo, Maria de, 32
Trump International, 60
Turbo, Tumo, 132–33
Two Boots, 89
Two-spot guide to spectating, 109

Ugali, 44, 47
Uncle George's, 93
Undulation profile of NYCM, 129–30
Union Square Café, 91
United Nations, 156
Upper East Side
   description of, 54, 55–56
   dining, recovery, 138
   running in, 69–70
Upper West Side
   description of, 54
   dining, recovery, 138–40
   running in, 68–69
UPS bags, 104
Uptown Manhattan, 54
Urban Ventures, 61
Urine color and water drinking, 42

V (interval training at VO2), 35
Van Cortlandt Park Cross-Country Races, 77, 164
Vanderbilt Y, 61
Van Hest, Greg, 32
Vaseline for chafing, 104, 106
Vaux, Calvert, 70, 145
Vegetarians, 46
Verazzano-Narrows Bridge, 97, 113, 121, 124, 130
Veterans of New York City Marathon, 24
Vo, Kiet, 67
Volunteering at NYCM, 28–29
V&T Pizzeria, 89

Wadsworth athletes' village, 103, 104
Waitz, Grete, 11, 12, 13, 14, 126, 133, 140–42, 161
Wakiihuri, Douglas, 14, 39, **39**, 98
Waking up, race day, 98
Walken, Christopher, 162
Walking
   alternating with running, 4
   recovery and, 135, 136, 137
"Wall," hitting the, 122, 126
Warmup
   race day and, 99–100, 106
   running and, 4, 35
Warriors' Tomb on the Plain of Marathon, xiv
Warwick, 60
Washington Heights, 55
Washington Square, 51
Water Club, The, 92
Water drinking
   race and planning, 119, 131–34
   recovery and, 136
   training and, 33, 34, 41–42, 43, 46

Water station workers (volunteers), 28
Water therapy for recovery, 136, 137
Weather
   clothing and, 3, 100–101, 106, 128–29
   NYCM and, 10, 14, 15, 19, 128–29
   training and, 33
Web sites
   NYC links, 176–77
   NYCM, 21
   running-related, 175–76
   travel accommodations, 61
Welch, Priscilla, 13, 162
West, Mae, 121
Westchester County running, 79
Westlund, Marielle, 134
West (odd-numbered streets), 52
West Side, 51, 63–64
West Side Y, 61
Wheelchair assistance, 97
Wheelchair division, NYCM, 22, 105
Willis Avenue Bridge, 113, 122, 126–27, 130
Winning margins (closest), NYCM, 164–65
WNBC, 108
Women runners
   elite women in NYCM, 104, 105
   facts/figures of NYCM, 9–19, 161–65
   nutrition for, 46
   NYCM start, 9
Wright, Frank Lloyd, 123
"Wrong-Way Silva," 15, 165

XT (cross-training), 35

Yatich, Mark, 46
Yellow number family reunion area, 124
YMCA, 61
Yo! (NYC speak), 89